Other Books Authored by Dr. John Halmaghi

Our Dental Office Manual: Policies, Processes, Procedures.

The Handbook Of Employment Policies: A Guide To Managing Office Personnel.

Do It Yourself Office Management Program

Before graduating from dental school at Michigan in 1988 Dr. "John" was actively involved in the management of four medical offices. After graduation he completed a GPR at Medical College of Ohio. Soon after, he joined a large group practice in Detroit where he helped open and manage two high volume dental offices. In 1990 he opened his first "scratch" practice, which quickly grew into the top 5%. In 1994 he sold this practice and opened another "scratch" practice which became a multi-million dollar business. In 2016 he sold this practice and took time off to enjoy his life and manage his real estate business. In 2020, he opened another scratch practice. He is currently practicing at this practice in Walled Lake, MI. He enjoys TMJ Headache treatment, cosmetics, orthodontics, reconstructive prosthodontics, endodontics, and cosmetics. Dr. "John," unlike many other authors and speakers, keeps an open door to all practitioners and invites you to stop by anytime for a visit. Dr John has also owned and operated 4 other profitable non-dental businesses and he truly enjoys buying, organizing, and selling businesses.

The material contained in this book may not be duplicated, copied, or reproduced in any fashion without express written consent of the author and publisher. You are advised to seek and consult local professionals concerning any legal, clinical, or professional advice. This book is protected by Copyright Law. The author and respective owners of this book cannot assume any responsibility or liability for the use and interpretation of any information contained within. The information contained in this book is based on "hands-on" experience, as well as knowledge accumulated through contacts with professionals. The reader is also advised to reference medical and dental textbooks in regard to possible complications, interferences, contraindications, and side-effects of all recommended drugs and supplies.

Copyright 2020, John Halmaghi

1935 N Pontiac Trail

Walled Lake, MI 48390

BALANCING THE CRITICAL ELEMENTS...

WHAT THEY DIDN'T TEACH YOU IN DENTAL SCHOOL!

Dr. John S. Halmaghi

copyright 2021

TABLE OF CONTENTS

INTRODUCTION 5
CHAPTER 1 THE NEW GRADUATE - WET EARS AND SLOW HANDS 9
CHAPTER 2 FINDING A JOB 12
CHAPTER 3 WHAT TO FOCUS ON (AFTER DENTAL SCHOOL) 14
CHAPTER 4 SETTING YOUR WORKING SCHEDULE AND SERVING MAINSTREAM AMERICA 19
CHAPTER 5 PRACTICE MADE PERFECT 26
CHAPTER 6 BURN-OUT AND STRESS 32
CHAPTER 7 YOUR GOALS AND PLANS 50
CHAPTER 8 TO BE OR NOT TO BE 62
CHAPTER 9 FINANCES/MONEY 69
CHAPTER 10 STAFF RELATIONS 80
CHAPTER 11 COMMON-SENSE EXPERTISE 86
CHAPTER 12 STOP - A WORD ABOUT EXPERTS 88
CHAPTER 13 COMMUNICATION/HUMAN RELATIONS 91
CHAPTER 14 THE INITIAL PATIENT APPOINTMENT 100
CHAPTER 15 THE PATIENT CASE PRESENTATION (YOU NEVER GET A SECOND CHANCE TO MAKE A FIRST IMPRESSION) 105
CHAPTER 16 TREATMENT PLANNING 116
CHAPTER 17 INSURANCE/COLLECTIONS 119
CHAPTER 18 COLLECTING YOUR MONEY 132
CHAPTER 19 BROKEN APPOINTMENTS, BROKEN HEARTS 138
CHAPTER 20 THE SPECIALTY ZONE 147
CHAPTER 21 OVERCOMING FEAR 149
CHAPTER 22 PEDODONTICS 155
CHAPTER 23 EMERGENCY CARE 157
CHAPTER 24 CLINICAL BASICS 161
CHAPTER 25 THE RUBBER DAM 163
CHAPTER 26 CARIES REMOVAL 166
CHAPTER 27 POST-OP SENSITIVITY 168
CHAPTER 28 RESTORATIVE DENTAL WORK 173
CHAPTER 29 ROOT CANALS 179
CHAPTER 30 CORES/BUILD-UPS 185
CHAPTER 31 CROWNS/PROSTHETICS 188
CHAPTER 32 EXTRACTIONS 199
CHAPTER 33 PERIO 202
CHAPTER 34 TMJ (TMD) 206
CHAPTER 35 OCCLUSION 212
CHAPTER 36 DENTURES/PARTIALS 215
CHAPTER 37 ESTHETICS 220
CHAPTER 38 ALL-PORCELAIN CROWNS AND VENEERS 224
Q & A 228
DR JOHN'S TOP TEN LIST 241

INTRODUCTION

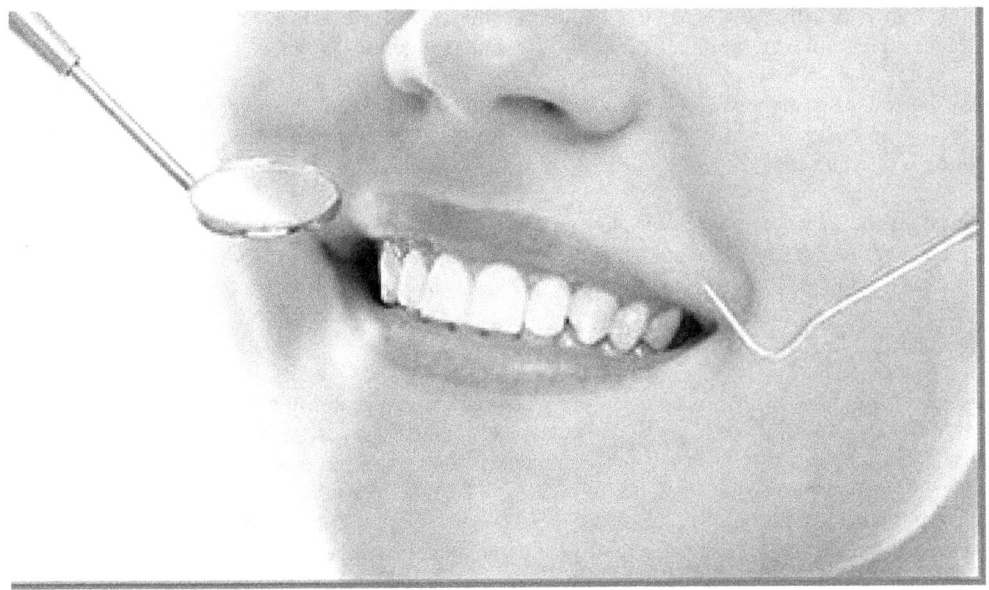

In a dental profession full of paper, experts, magazines, books, online guides and journals some of the best ideas and suggestions are never published. The professionals who are successful usually do not have the time to talk or write about their achievements. The dental marketplace does not support great works of writing because the professionals with the most to say are usually too busy to spend their time writing. So, comes this book. Written out of a pure desire to expand my hobbies, this work is a labor of love. It was not written with an intent to be a best-seller or money maker. It was written out of the pure interest to share my learnings, ideas, and experiences with dental graduates and other practitioners.

The dental profession boasts one of the highest "disenchantment" rates among all of the professions. Sad as it may be, according to recent surveys, 65% of today's practitioners are regretful of the choice that they made to become dentists. An even larger percentage of practitioners earn incomes that are less than the earnings of common tradesmen. These statistics are never discussed in dental school. Recent dental graduates are being thrown into the "lion's den" without guidance. The dental field forgets about its students and its future. The outcome usually becomes a scary statistic. Nobody cares about the new kid on the block. The dental profession lives up to the "dog eat dog" mentality, as many practitioners scramble to find patients and income, while being overly competitive with their colleagues and negligent of the profession's future - the young practitioner. This handbook is dedicated to the recent graduate/practitioner who is ready to take the "plunge" into the sea of dentistry.

The real world of dentistry is often filled with disillusionment, anger, and frustration. This author hopes to change the reader's outlook and attitude towards his/her profession. This book will help you get on track towards a profitable and enjoyable future in the dental profession. It is the scope of this book to help you achieve a better financial and professional future by discussing the various topics and ways of developing your personal and clinical skills.

This book is also intended to give advice to the established practitioner who may have forgotten about some basic aspects of being a profitable and successful dentist. Sometimes a refresher course is all you need.

Leaving dental school is often an unpredictable experience, as most students quickly come to realize that there are few helping hands waiting for them. It does not take long to figure out that there is a major change of pace as you step forward into the profession of dentistry. The "motherly" nurture of the dental school curriculum is quickly replaced by the reality of the obstacles that face most practicing dentists.

Usually the hardest aspect of entering the work force is your ability to make decisions and set goals. This book will provide you with some eye-opening facts and suggestions that will ease the obstacles and hardships facing your future goals. Once you have some practical information about the dental profession your future goals will become easier to reach. This book will help open up your eyes and your mind. It will help to reduce the number of mistakes that you could possibly make during the infant stage of your career, and it will help to propel you into success at a faster pace. A lot of the information provided herein has been attained over the years from my personal and professional experience. I hope that some of the mistakes that I made during the early part of my career can be avoided by you - the reader. This book will provide you with the required knowledge necessary to avoid making costly errors and poor decisions. In turn, your financial and professional growth will flower at a faster and less burdensome pace.

According to the ADA in 1996 (when I released the first version of this book) there were over 150,000 practicing dentists and approximately 70,000 dental practices in the US. 10% of these practices were considered large operations, employing at least 5 associates and over 25 staff members. The other 90% of practices averaged one dentist with 3 staff members. Today, less than 77% of practices are owned by dentists while coporate dentistry has grown over 25% in recent years alone. There are now over 200,000 dentists in our country. The shift towards corporate dentistry will continue. The average gross revenues of today's practice is averaging $771,000. Overhead expense averages range from 50% to as high as 80%. Bread and butter dentistry is still the mainstem of services being provided. The current net income of young dental practitioners (1-5 years of out dental school) is approximately $150,000. For every five years in increase of seniority, the net income improves by about $25,000, reaching a plateau of $250,000 for experienced (15 or more years in practice) dentists. This book will help you reach the top income plateau within the next 5 years.

If you have picked up this book and you are currently one of the lucky few to own your practice, then join us for a look at some basic points of patient and practice management that you may have forgotten about.

When I began to write this book I entitled it "The New Graduate - A Guide To Becoming A Profitable Dentist." After I had a few colleagues review the book I decided to change the name. My scope in writing this book was to help direct the new graduate towards a happy, fulfilling, and prosperous career. It is also meant to help established practitioners and practice owners review some basic fundamentals that are crucial to surviving in a competitive market. Learning to balance the critical elements of dentistry, along with your personal life, is the only way to achieve this goal. Written from a practical viewpoint, this book is purposeful and helpful at any level of the dental career.

This book should help you recognize the fact that there is more to dentistry than working on the dentition. For the practitioner who realizes that dentistry is a people business, and not a tooth business, you are light years ahead. Patients come to you with a need. You may meet this need through providing dental services, but you will not develop your professional and personal goals by simply doing so. You must learn to meet your patient's dental and emotional needs in order to become successful and profitable. This book will help teach you how to communicate with patients and provide quality dental care in order to meet those needs.

As dentists we have always been scared of insurance companies and their low reimbursements. All practitioners feel that net income is decreasing while expenses are sky-rocketing. Employers and employees are signing up for PPOs at alarming rates. Dentists are faced with the reality of having to join these plans in order to pay their bills. Although this reality is certainly not amusing, a lot of practitioners are forgetting to look at some basic facts.. Dental schools are graduating nearly 50% female dentists whose professional life expectancy is less than 10 to 15 years. At the same time, the increased consumption of bottled spring water and high-fructose colas is still causing dental disease. A prediction that I made back in 1996 was due to my fear that we would enter a crisis of quality dental care has in this country. Today's dental care is severely deprived of quality. I spend more time fixing dental work from other offices than anything else I do. If you are ready and willing to improve your people and clinical skills, you have nothing to worry about. Wait and reap the benefits. Let the assembly line dentists worry about corporate profits. Develop your personal and clinical skills and patients will beat a path to your door.

This book will focus on those things that will help you achieve what you want out of dentistry. First, realize that....

The common trait of a successful person is the ability to communicate with others in order to gain trust and acceptance.

Once this happens, the exchange of services for money becomes a simple stepping stone. Hopefully, after reading this book, you will realize that in order to treat your patients adequately and profitably you must learn to communicate effectively.

<u>Author's note:</u> at the end of each chapter I have tried to include some ideas, suggestions, and para-phrases of wisdom. Take your time and read these slowly. Try to adapt one of these principles daily into your life. Let's start here:

<u>VISION:</u> **The Ability To Look Beyond Your Own Back Yard!**

<u>PERSEVERANCE:</u> **The Person Who Removes A Mountain Begins By Carrying Small Stones!**

<u>FAITH:</u> **The Ability To Follow Your Opinion In Search Of Your Beliefs.**

<u>OBSTACLES:</u> **You Won't See Them Unless You Take Your Eyes Off Of Your Goals.**

<u>HOPE:</u> **It Makes The World!**

SUCCESS IS ATTITUDE!

DON'T WAIT FOR TOMORROW, TODAY IS YOUR FUTURE!

CHAPTER 1
THE NEW GRADUATE - WET EARS AND SLOW HANDS

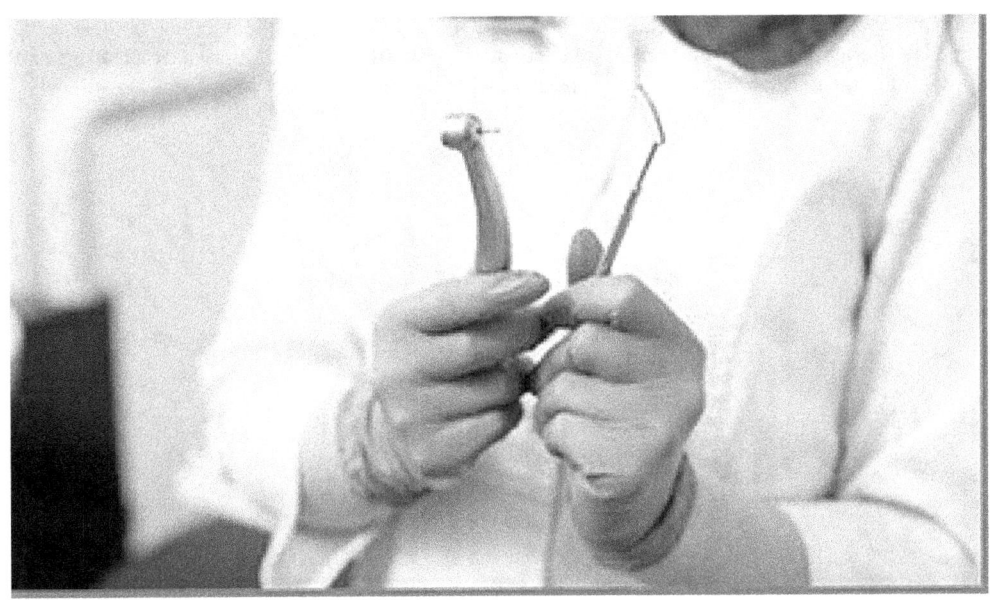

When I graduated from dental school at Michigan, I entered a GPR program. This was by far the most educative part of my dental career. I learned all aspects of clinical dentistry and received a lot of background in medicine. I wish that all dental schools would make a GPR program a post-graduate requirement. You are simply not ready to make waves into private practice upon graduating from dental school, whether it is in your own practice or as an associate. Your skills are not developed, your motor coordination is slow, and your diagnostic capabilities are far from adequate. I don't mean to burst your bubble, or demean your abilities, but I know from observing my fellow classmates and myself, that upon graduating from school, your skills as a dentist are "infantile" and for the most part - poor. Michalengelo did not paint the Sistine without years of practice and experience. Einstein did not produce the theory of relativity without years of research.

Young dentists need more than five years to become knowledgeable and skilled practitioners. Some need nine lives!

The latter part of this book will detail some clinical aspects of dentistry that will help you get started towards developing above average dental skills and abilities.

For those of you who are debating whether to open up your own place right from the start, I have one simple piece of advice: <u>wait at least two years!</u> Work in a large group practice, if you cannot get a GPR, or seek a relationship with an established practitioner. Over 65% of practicing dentists are currently regretting their careers. If these facts are not enough to scare you out of deciding to open up your own practice, then keep reading.

This book will help you decide whether you have the desire, the skills, and the attitude to go forth with your dream. Best of all, this book will help you get ready for being on your own someday. **Being a dentist is a challenge in its own, without the extra burden of running and managing a business.** For the doctor willing to tackle both jobs, good luck and good reading!!!

TELL THE TRUTH!

DON'T DO THINGS YOU DISLIKE.

MAKE A POSITIVE DIFFERENCE IN THE LIVES OF OTHERS.

LIVE TO GROW AND IMPROVE.

SMELL THE ROSES.

DON'T CONCENTRATE ON WHAT YOU CANNOT DO.

THE HARDER YOU WORK, THE LUCKIER YOU GET.

WORK FOR A PURPOSE OTHER THAN MONEY.

DON'T JUDGE PEOPLE.

CHAPTER 2
FINDING A JOB

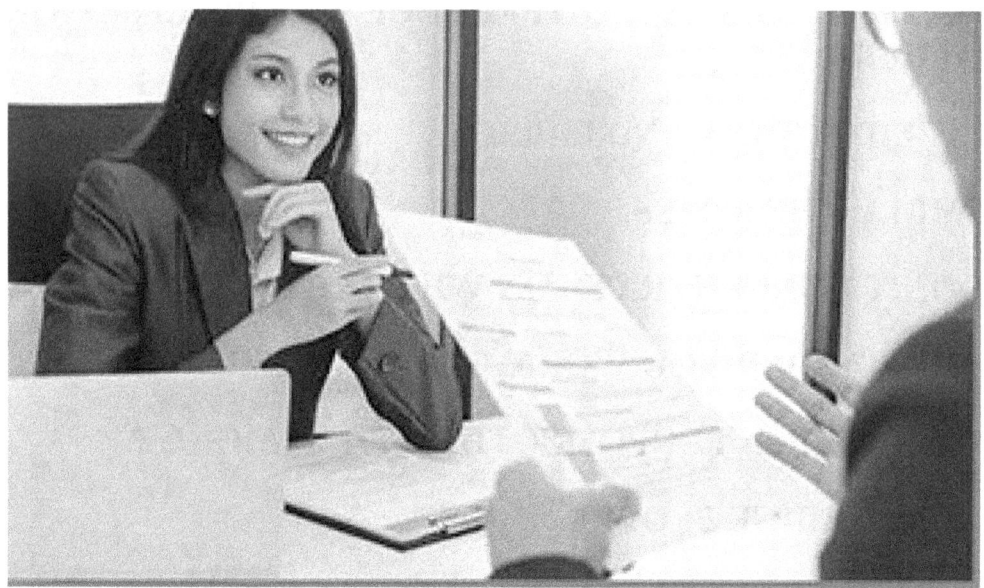

The first thing you will have to do as you step foot out of school is to find a job. No kiddin'!

Graduating students who do not have family members to provide guidance and opportunity must start searching and beating the path. Your state dental association monthly publication is usually the best source of information for finding the appropriate employment opportunity. Search these listings monthly. Maintain membership in the ADA, and its component societies, during your first three years after graduation.

Begin to send out your professional resume to all potential employers. I like to receive resumes from students, especially when I am **not** advertising for any positions. I keep all resumes for future reference. You may want to consider sending out your resume to all dentists in the area that you wish to work in. Do a simple Google search and see which practices pop up first in the business listings. Contact these offices/doctors personally by the telephone, and follow up with a mailed resume. You never know when someone is going to be looking for an associate or partner. Although you may not have the option of working exactly where you would like during your first few years of practice, you should make it your goal to practice where you are needed. **It is not important to make your office location close to your home.** <u>The key is to serve those people/patients that need you.</u>

Remember the following when sending out your resume: **state your ability to be be able to perform profitable dentistry and build the practice patient base.** Most employers do not care about your big accomplishments or research projects that you completed in school. They want to know what you can bring to the practice in terms of future financial potential and patient growth. Send a letter, with the resume, that indicates exactly what you can do clinically and practically. Forget about your awards and diplomas. Market yourself as a businessperson and able clinician. The past does not equal the future. State something like the following:

"I am sending this resume to your attention. If you are looking for an energetic and self-motivated associate, please keep me in mind. I have excellent bed-side manners, as well as knowledge of what it takes to produce profitable, quality dental care. I am willing to help you manage the small problems in your office, take your after-hour emergencies, and provide your patients with efficient and thorough dental care. I also hope to help you build your practice through internal marketing, staff management/training, and any other possible avenues of promotions. I am open to working late evenings and Saturdays. I can handle more than one patient at a time and I possess great communication skills that help me to motivate patients into accepting necessary treatment. I enjoy treatment planning crowns, bridges, and esthetic dentistry. I am skilled at the following areas of dentistry: _____."

Spend at least two months researching the market and acquainting yourself with the practitioners in your area. It is also helpful to seek the advice of your local dental supply company. Many of these companies provide lists of practitioners who are looking to hire new graduates. Do not be alarmed if most of your job offers come from "large" practices where staff changes are as common as weather patterns in Illinois. These large practice settings are conducive to developing your skills and giving you some knowledge on management and marketing. The experienced practitioners are usually not going to hire new graduates. Don't let this disappoint you! Someday, when you become one of those high-profile, quality dentists, you will also not consider hiring a recent graduate.

STAY IN SHAPE

EAT RIGHT

GET A PHYSICAL...

ONE CANNOT FUNCTION EFFICIENTLY IF THEY ARE NOT TAKING CARE OF THEIR MOST IMPORTANT ASSET: THEIR HEALTH!

CHAPTER 3
WHAT TO FOCUS ON (AFTER DENTAL SCHOOL)

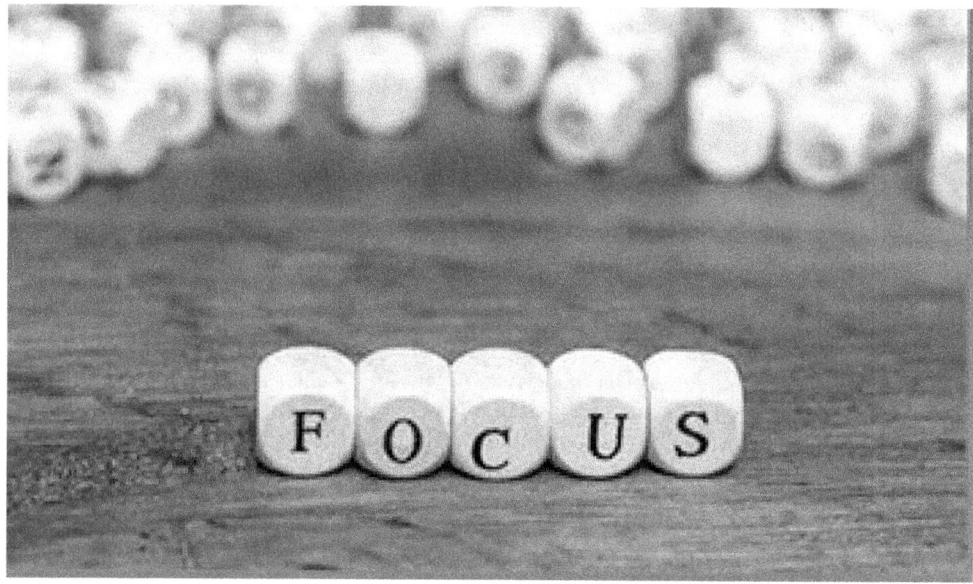

Your main goals during the first three years of practicing dentistry are to develop your clinical skills, learn some aspects of business management, and improve your communication skills.

Don't be afraid to accept a position in a low income area where the need for dental services exceeds the supply.

Although you may want to work in an upscale office, where the waiting room has Italian ceramic tile and the operatories are overstocked, your skills will develop much faster by providing bread and butter dentistry in an area where the demand for your services is high. Be open to providing services for Medicaid and low-income patients. You will gain an immense amount of clinical knowledge and experience. You will also receive a lot of gratitude from patients who will respect your care. You can earn a comfortable income while gaining this experience. However, you should concentrate on improving your personal and clinical skills during your first five years of practice rather than worrying about how much money you make.

After I graduated from dental school, I began a pseudo-partnership with a multiple location organization. I was providing dental care to patients in low income areas. I took advantage of my situation by sharpening my skills and performing a lot of dental procedures. When some of the services that I wanted to perform were not covered by "insurance," I developed my skills by offering patients gratuitous dentistry. I performed many molar root canals, at no charge. In the process I gained a wealth of experience. I also performed a lot of surgical extractions to improve my skills and speed. Don't overlook such an opportunity for improvement. I see too many graduates developing an "ostrich" attitude. They want to treat only fee for service patients between 9 and 5. These birds often wonder why they're making garbage man wages and re-doing a lot of their sub-standard work.

I have hired many associates in previous years who lacked the determination to become profitable practitioners. Some of these recent graduates even wanted to be home by 5 p.m. to be with their families. Although I admire family dedication, the young practitioner must do everything possible to go out of their way to work hard and improve their clinical skills. If you want to cover all bases (good job, comfortable pay, ample patients) you must develop your clinical and personal skills by going out of your way. This includes the necessity to make yourself available during evening hours and Saturdays. At the same time it also includes the requirement to stay busy by accepting all types of patients that will help you to **practice, practice, practice**. More on this topic in the next chapter.

In a recent study performed by Planned Marketing Associates it was found that 30% of the dentists perform over 70% of the dental business in our country.

That means that 60,000 dentists are busy doing dental work, while 140,000 are slow, lazy, and lethargic.

Choose, early in your career, which group you want to be part of. You have invested an immense amount of time and money in earning your dental degree. Don't let it go to waste. Get your gloves wet and just do it!

The success of any dentist, whether young or "mature," depends upon solid clinical skills and excellent personal demeanor. In order to develop your abilities as an excellent practitioner you must understand that this takes time and practice. The capability to provide excellent dental care does not happen overnight. You must practice, learn, observe, practice, learn, observe, etc. **The learning curve of dentistry is infinite**. The more you do, the faster you perform. It's like a video-game. Play it once, you feel like a fool. Play it ten times, you get past level 1. Play it a hundred times, you can become decent. Play it a thousand times, you can do it with your eyes closed. This is true for you clinical development as well as your personal improvement.

Recent graduates are like greyhounds waiting to shoot out of the gate. They can't wait to get out in the real world to make some money and show everyone just how much they learned in dental school. Take a deep breath, because you are not going to change the wheel! There is a narrow-minded belief amongst graduates that they don't want any supervision or any dentists "looking over their shoulders" as they begin to practice dentistry. This attitude is self defeating to practitioners who desire to get started on the right track towards professional development! Welcome the opportunity for a mentor (senior dentist) to give you insight, input, and evaluation of your dental work. Seek the help and advice of such a mentor, at all times, during your career.

There will always be a dentist who is better than you. There will always be someone a step ahead of you. Find these people during your career. Don't be afraid to have your crown margins evaluated. Welcome a caries removal check, once in a while. Have an open mind in regard to criticism and input. Most important, become active in study groups and continuing education.

Once you realize that it takes time and hard work to develop your professional skills, half of the battle is won. The other half is to be patient and allow time for this self-improvement to take place. Of course, it is important for you to always seek seminar and continuing education programs, in order to keep up with the latest developments in dentistry. Concentrate your efforts towards learning basic clinical dentistry for the first three years. You can expand your knowledge of advanced dentistry **after you master general dentistry.**

You must constantly keep current of the latest developments in dentistry. A lot of the procedures that you were taught in dental school are what I call "Mrs. Field's Recipes." The basic procedures that you learned in school are procedures that have been proven over the years. There is absolutely nothing wrong with performing these procedures, however there are constant innovations and new ways to skin the cat. Once you have mastered the dental school basics, you must open up your eyes to the new techniques and products available on the market. There are many seminars and material available to you. You will quickly become bombarded with a lot of marketing on this stuff. Wee-whack your way through some of this material and pick out the gems.

Visit the following websites for CE:
www.agd.org
www.dentalcare.com
www.glidewelldental.com
www.ada.org
www.cezoom.com

Always look for free CE, but don't forget that self-study online courses CE can only count for a certain number of requirements per your state licensure. The Chicago Midwinter is one of the finest meetings in the country. You can get most of your CE requirements done at this meeting.

Your state dental association meeting (and ADA Annual Session) is usually one of the best places to attend a variety of seminars. Call your component, or district society, for more information about these and other upcoming speakers and events. These meetings are usually the best bang for your buck. The meetings are also a great way to meet other practitioners, and exchange information. It is also helpful to attend local and county dental society meetings.

Remember to maintain a current address with all of the dental publications that are available to you, at no charge. These monthly journals have a vast amount of clinical and management material. Most of the articles and information is written by the same speakers and experts who charge hundreds of dollars for their seminars. Take advantage of the publications and their contents. Make sure to allow at least one day per month to review these journals. When reading journal articles make notes of the parentheses items. Authors will list the manufacturers of the materials and supplies that they use for the procedures described. Some of these materials may not be available through your local vendors and you may want to call the manufacturer directly. You should also make a habit of observing the ads for new dental materials and products. Today's innovation is tomorrow's obsolence! Always strive to stay ahead of your competition by researching new techniques, materials, and products.

Pay attention to offers for books and videos. Many seminars can be purchased at a fraction of the cost of attending a seminar in person. You Tube University will always have a ton of education.

Before discussing any clinical topics and strategies we are going to cover some of the more important aspects of becoming successful and profitable: setting goals and improving your communication skills. A practitioner that lacks the ability to identify, set and achieve his/her goals is like a ship sailing without a compass and rudder. This same practitioner must also develop excellent communication skills in order to achieve their goals. We are going to spend a few chapters on these topics.

The rest of this book is therefore going to center around setting your goals, improving your communication process, and sharpening your clinical skills. The practitioner who is willing to master these skills will become efficient, happy, and profitable.

WHEN YOU JUDGE OTHERS YOU ARE REFLECTING YOUR OWN WEAKNESSES.

TAKE RISKS.

FORGIVE AND FORGET.

YOU CAN ONLY BE AS HAPPY AS YOU MAKE UP YOUR MIND TO BE.

CHOOSE TO LOSE BEFORE CHOOSING TO WIN DISHONESTLY.

DON'T ASKY "WHY," ASK "WHY NOT?"

TREASURE LOVE ABOVE ALL ELSE.

CHAPTER 4
SETTING YOUR WORKING SCHEDULE AND SERVING MAINSTREAM AMERICA

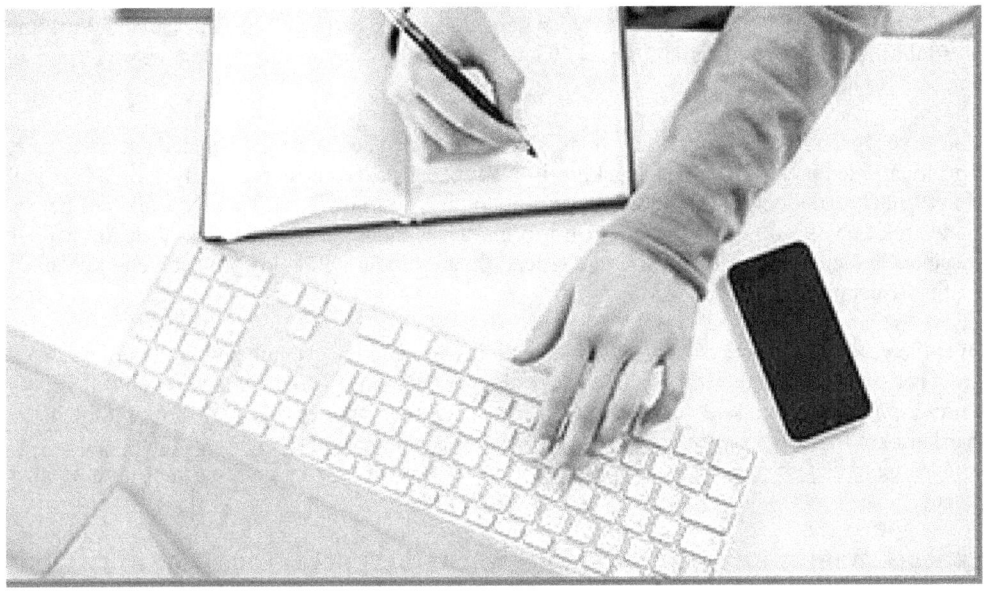

How you decide to set your work schedule will affect your entire career. Dental school curriculum no longer controls your life, so it is up to you to decide how you want to work. You must take many factors into consideration:

1. Number of days to work per week.
2. Hours and times of day to work per week.
3. The time of day that you are most efficient and productive.
4. What type of work you enjoy doing most.
5. What type of work you would rather refer.
6. How fast you can perform various procedures.

In order to gain clinical knowledge and master various techniques, you must have adequate time **to perform, experiment, learn, adjust, and improve.** You have to gain control of your schedule in order to be able to do so. I love to read articles by well known experts who equate scheduling to inanimate objects and Olympic obstacles. What a total joke! Scheduling is done to serve those human beings that we call patients. It should not be designed strictly for profit and high production.

Effective scheduling leads to profit, happiness, learning, and goal achievement as long as it takes into account the fact that you are performing dental care to serve your patients to the best of your abilities.

How you work is up to you, and nobody else. Some of your choices will be based on family and personal reasons, but you also have to consider the schedule of your patients and your staff. Most of all, you have to realize that you are helping people and making a difference in their lives, not in your pocketbook. You must stick to your guns during the early part of your career. Work the schedule that fits your goals and needs, while taking into account the reason why you are in practice - <u>to help people!</u>

You have received excellent training in all areas of dentistry, except for advanced specialty care. You must attempt to develop your skills in all type of procedures, especially the "bread and butter" stuff: endodontics, periodontics, prosthodontics, restorative, oral surgery, and aesthetics. You cannot be afraid to perform and learn to master as many basic principles of dental care as possible. The more you can perform and repeat, the more you will enjoy your job and become a profitable dentist.

Over the years I have noticed that my "best" patients come in the evening and on Saturdays. So, I stay open during those times. Of course, I am always available for emergencies, even if it is only a prescription phone call. My associate helps to expand my practice hours by working the hours that I am not there. <u>Do not be brain-washed by experts who tell you to set your hours and not let your patients dictate when you should work.</u> This is a great way of inviting them into another practice.

Patients want you to be available when they need you, not when it is convenient for you.

To have a productive, efficient, and non-stressful schedule you must sit down with your appointment coordinator and implement a schedule with guidelines that meet your practice philosophy. How much time you want to spend for each procedure is totally up to you, but you must time yourself and constantly strive to increase your speed and decrease the appointment times. If you find yourself constantly running behind schedule, then you must sit down with the front desk persons and "iron" things out. I am a true believer in working fast and efficiently. I despise running behind and making patients wait. I always let my front desk know how much time I request for the patient's next appointment because I know exactly what I want to accomplish and I know how long it takes me to do so. If I run behind it is either because of an emergency or some unforeseen problems.

Early in my career, many unforeseen, "rookie problems" stemmed from inexperience. These problems slowed me down. After gaining more experience, these unpredictabilities became rare. I have learned to control them and prepare for them through **pro-active thinking, planning and**

constant self-improvement. Time yourself every day and see how long it takes you to complete different procedures. Then work on speeding yourself up without sacrificing quality. Learn to eliminate set-backs and problems through education and experience. Those long, curved endodontic mesial canals should not slow you down once you learn to master them and control your technique. The ill-fitting matrix band should not be a hassle once you learn to treatment plan more crowns and onlays.

Read the following sentence ten times: Profitability comes from full quadrant dentistry performed without remakes and problems.

You cannot perform this kind of dentistry if you have to pogo-stick-it from room to room all day long. I practiced jumping jack dentistry for many years, until I ended up in physical therapy for dislocated thoracic vertebrae. Although in some high-volume practices you must perform this kind of dentistry to keep your paycheck, it is a sure way to early retirement or burn-out. High volume dentistry may be profitable, but it is not enjoyable and self-fulfilling, over the lifespan of your professional career. If you can learn to communicate with your patients you do not need to be in this type of environment. Even if you accept a lot of PPOs you do not need to jog between operatories. Worry about developing your reputation through caring, gentle care...the finances will follow in later years. Patients will choose alternative treatments that are not covered by insurance: whitening, veneers, TMJ therapy, implants, Invisalign, etc.

In my first practice I used to schedule up to 50 patients per day. We accepted Medicaid and some other low fee programs. To stay profitable we performed as much basic dentistry as we could, running from room to room all day long. Guess what we lacked in this type of environment? You got it: communication. In my present office, we schedule according to patient needs. Some days we may only see 2 patients that need 5 crowns each and other days we may see 10 patients that each need single crowns. It is rare to schedule more than 12 patients. Currently, I perform mainly TMJ/Headache Treatment, cosmetics, Invisalign, root canals, cores, crowns, and multiple unit prosthodontics. I do more of this type of treatment than ever before because I take the time to diagnose it, treatment plan it, recommend it, and motivate it. Again, communication, communication, communication. If I was running from room to room doing bits and pieces, how could I spend the time to communicate with new patients? Of course, I have gained trust and respect with many patients that have been loyal customers for many years.

Early in my career, It took me some time to realize that I was becoming ineffective with my communication process with many of my patients, especially the ones that had good coverages and steady incomes. When I decided to restructure my schedule, I found more time for communication. Consequently, I find myself working less and less, while producing more and more. I concentrate on the high-fee procedures and I gain case acceptance through effective communication. My schedule is drastically different now then it was years ago because it is controlled by myself and the type of procedures that I enjoy doing. I did not have this choice when I was getting my feet wet. It took me a few years to reach this stage of my career. Many of those early Medicaid and capitation patients are now paying cash for my services. And I am still grateful for the opportunity that I had to improve my skills.

At my office, quadrant dentistry is the only way I appoint patients. Single tooth dentistry is done at recalls.

The average length of my appointments is 90 minutes. The goal is multiple unit restorative or root canal(s), core(s), crown(s). Multiple procedures performed on the same patient...gently, esthetically, and functionally.

Emergencies are also top priorities. They are excellent practice builders, the average extraction takes no more than 15 minutes, and many end up into the 90 minute brackets (root canal, core crown, perio....the works - if I have time).

New patients receive 60 minutes, out of which approximately 10 minutes is undisturbed time with myself. Recalls are seen for no more than 40 minutes. Adjustments, deliveries, bites, try-ins, consultations, and other short procedures are scheduled at random, for less than 15 minutes. Periodontal procedures are scheduled according to the needs of the patient.

In order to be able to run a smooth schedule you must be in control of it. This means constant communication with the front desk. Not a single patient is appointed without my instructions and directives. I tell the front desk exactly how much time I want for each and every patient appointment. In a profitable practice, minutes count.

To begin a profitable and joyful day you must start by taking control of your schedule and reviewing ahead.

- What problems will there be today?
- What difficult patients are we going to encounter?
- Were all necessary pre-meds given?
- Were smokers prescribed Valium and Benadryl?
- Have TMJ patients been screened and treated before restorative work?
- Is sedation or Nitrous necessary for anyone?
- Were premeds called in?
- Have treatment plans been completed?
- Have financial responsibilities been explained?
- What are we going to delegate to the assistants?
- Are all lab cases completed and available?
- Do any of the patients have a history of broken appointments and can we fill the schedule in case of no-shows?

These are simple questions that you must ask and answer before the beginning of the day. I call this brainstorming session "The Morning Huddle." Without it you cannot gain control of your schedule.

To increase your speed and improve the efficiency of your schedule, here are a few more helpful ideas:

1. For New Patients: try to do a cleanng unless you diagnose perio problems. If there is gingivitis or beginning periodontitis, do not pick up the scalers. Do a quick debridement, oral hygiene instructions, education, give brochures, and re-appoint if the patient seems enthusiastic about completing treatment.
2. Get emergencies in the same day. Prescribe if you are behind, or take the extra ten minutes to relieve pain. Develop a new relationship with that patient.
3. Learn endodontics and perform it. Most endo can be performed in under 30 minutes and in one appointment.
4. Use modern equipment, especially ultrasonics. Use multiple handpieces and avoid changing burs.
5. Delegate, within state laws.
6. Do not work in a pool of blood. Optimize periodontal health before you begin restorative, especially interproximally. Bleeding gums will drive you crazy and diminish the quality of your work.
7. Use DryShield or a Rubber Dam or Isolite. If you cannot use either then at least use the clamps with cotton rolls. Never remove amalgam without such aids. You will get mercury toxicity from removing amalgams!
8. Work with two assistants
9. Learn to use "anesthetic time" to do small procedures. Hygiene checks, emergencies, deliveries, adjustments, etc. can be done while the quadrant patient is getting numb.
10. Review finances at each and every appointment. Do not pick up the instruments until you are certain that the patient understands their financial responsibilities.
11. Organize your tray and/or drawer set-ups. When you are going to be performing a certain procedure the entire set-up, including all instruments and supplies, should be available with a simple grab. Visit your local hardware or department store and purchase kitchen tray/storage organizers and assemble your set-ups if you do not have enough drawers in operatories. Do not be cheap when it comes to ordering extra instruments and supplies. The less motions you have to make to set a room for a procedure, the more efficient you will be. At my old office, my crown and bridge set-ups were included in carpenter's boxes that had everything from mixing tips to retraction cord. My composite set-ups were placed in desk organizers that had partitions for all of the different shades and necessary supplies. My other set-ups are also designed to promote efficiency without running around looking for instruments. If you have ever worked in an operating room you know what organization and set-ups are. Today, every procedure has a drawer in the operatory and we now use Omnichroma so no need for multiple composite compules.
12. Clean and organize your front desk area. Have all necessary paperwork readily available. All forms and handouts should be stored on a server and easily accessible from any computer station for easy printing or signing.
13. Conduct weekly training sessions with employees. Do not be afraid to waste supplies and train your assistants. Delegated duties make you profitable and efficient.
14. Video-tape yourself during certain procedures and look for inefficiencies and wasted motions.

15. Stock all rooms adequately and equally. If one of your tray set-ups is missing a bur or other instrument it should be available in the operatory as a back-up. Do not waste time running around for supplies and instruments.
16. Teach all staff members about patient education and distributing brochures and having videos available for viewing.
17. Avoid making custom trays for single and double units.
18. Schedule variety...avoid sameness. Talk to your endodontist once in a while!
19. Keep evening and Saturday appointments open, even one day in advance. Many patients want those last minute appointments. I like to block off at least one hour on Mondays and Fridays for late-comers and/or emergencies. These slots do not get appointed until the last possible minute (usually the same day). You will find this to be a great way of having belated patients coming in for treatment. Keeping open slots in your schedule will allow you to see more emergencies and patients that like to do their Christmas shopping at the last minute. Since I brought up the holiday issue, you will find many patients wanting last minute appointments during the holidays in order to take advantage of their unused insurance benefits. Keep times available during this season and schedule your other patients later on.
20. Don't wreck your brain by using *goal and daily production* sheets that so many speakers advocate to help you reach daily money goals. This is garbage philosophy that is detrimental to positive activity, especially during times that uncontrollable situations prevent you from attaining the goals. Do what is right for your patients and keep a constantly busy schedule. Think about performing quality, quadrant dentistry. The production will be there. What would your patients think if they saw one of these charts in your office?

Profitability comes from honest, quality, full quadrant dentistry performed without remakes and problems.

It does not come from graphs and tables.

BE THE MOST ENTHUSIASTIC PERSON THAT YOU CAN BE

BE SPONTANEOUS

SAY "I CAN"

SAY "I WILL"

BE DETERMINED

MANAGE YOUR TIME

DON'T GET COMPLACENT

SLAP YOURSELF WHEN YOU THINK NEGATIVE THOUGHTS

DON'T BE AFRAID

MAKE OPPORTUNITIES, DON'T LOOK FOR THEM

JOBS HAVE NO FUTURE. THE FUTURE LIES IN THE WORKER

CHAPTER 5
PRACTICE MADE PERFECT

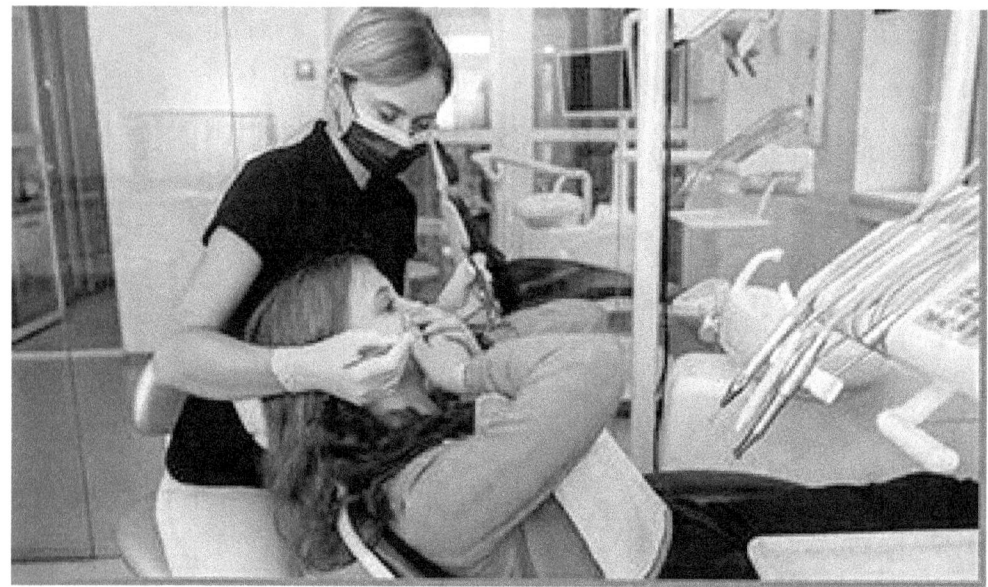

Practice makes perfect! Have you ever heard this wisdom before? If so, throw it out with your refuse. You, along with 100% of the population, will never be perfect. There is no such thing. Mistakes are necessary, perfection is only a word. In order to be efficient clinically you must practice to improve, not to be perfect.

A lot of dentists strive to achieve perfection without realizing that there is no such animal. If you fail to realize that you are human, and you do not allow for errors, you are going to be a miserable and non-profitable dentist/person.

Nothing in dentistry is life and death, except for a cardiac standstill.

Attempt to provide above average dental work to the best of your abilities. Accept mistakes and failures. Get out of the elitist attitude. One of my favorite jokes about dentists refers to forming an execution firing squad. If this group was being formed out of dentists they would all form a circle and not one would request a blank bullet. Dentists love to ridicule and find fault with the work of their fellow doctor. It is an inherent, and anal quality, that dentists are born with: I am better than the rest! I am perfect! Everyone else is an idiot! Get out of this mentality!

On the other hand, it is natural and healthy to admire the doctors who can provide quality dental care that includes many procedures other than basic dentistry. We all look up to the dentists who can perform implants, TMJ, oral surgery, orthodontics, etc. It is motivating to want to improve your skills and knowledge. It is unhealthy to demean your colleagues in a vain attempt to pedestal yourself. At the same time, you must realize that **your income and sanity will be achieved through optimal performance of bread/butter dentistry** (composites, crowns, bridges, extractions, dentures, cleanings, periodontics, and cosmetics). Specialized dental care is not going to make a huge difference in your future, <u>unless</u> you perform it on a <u>regular basis with quantitative numbers.</u>

A lot of dentists spend an immense amount of time developing their skills towards the specialties. By the time they learn these skills they come to realize that they should have spend their efforts trying to build their patient base and/or their practices with general procedures. Usually the time invested in trying to become the jack of all trades (master of none) is not worth the return. The time taken away from other activities ends up as a loss in later years.

This does not mean that you should not attempt to improve your dental skills. By all means, your future depends on improving your techniques and knowledge. Learn and improve yourself constantly. Just don't try to be everything to everyone at all times. Do what you enjoy! Do it right and do it fast!

To make money in any business you must do procedures that you can perform quickly and consistently. Trying to provide too many different services takes away from your ability to be fast and good. If you take a look at any manufacturing process, or even the fast food franchises, you will find that they make their profit by doing the same thing exceptionally well, over and over again. McDonald's would not try to make burritos, while Taco Bell would not attempt to make Big Macs. Either would lose money trying to copy the other. It is the same in dentistry. Provide basic services that you enjoy performing adequately, consistently, and quickly. Slowly, add other services if you so desire and see a need for your patients.

As you progress through your highway of dental learning you must start to evaluate the care that you enjoy providing. Dentistry is a very demanding profession. Providing services that you do not enjoy performing will only lead to burnout and stress. Don't become a part of the statistics. Provide care that you enjoy. Provide it professionally, ethically, and profitably. If you don't enjoy dentistry get out while you are young and do something else. Do something you enjoy!

A positive financial outlook awaits you once you understand that it takes time to become successful. As my father once told me, " It took me twenty years to become an overnight success." The oceans were build one drop at a time. Your goals will take time to reach.

As you are developing your career you have to work your butt off and you need to have an open attitude towards improving yourself before you can improve your financial portfolio. For most young graduates, this learning curve takes a minimum of five years. During this period of time you must have an open attitude towards treating all types of patients and performing all types of procedures, in order to get **experience and overcome the unpredictable events of your profession.** Welcome the chance to serve as many patients as possible while you are developing your skills, even if it means accepting managed care and capitation. After you build your reputation and develop your skills, you can worry about limiting the patients that you see, if that will still be possible. But at the beginning of your career you must work hard and develop your expertise.

When you decide to serve your patients you have to take into account your needs, as well as the needs of your patients. After 30 years of private practice, I still maintain three late evening and Saturday hours. My patients work, and I have to be available for them according to their schedule, not mine. Although it is rare that I work more than 30 hours per week, I try to be flexible and keep the office open according to the demand of my patients. I do not accept PPOs but my basic philosophy about low reimbursement programs is that you do not need to participate with them - as long as your chairs are full, during the times that you want to work. If your chairs are empty, then you have to seriously consider accepting plans that will bring patients into your office. While you are starting out you should remove the blindfolds and treat as many patients as possible. The more patients you can treat, in a relaxed and non-hurried manner, the more you will learn and improve your skills. Attempt to work a minimum of 40 hours per week during your first five years. Take the time to diagnose, perform, evaluate, and repeat as many procedures as possible while your clinical skills are developing. Remember the video-game comparison!

I receive many calls from recent graduates who ask my opinion about managed care and PPOs. Remember the golden rule: your patients don't know s--- about insurance. Unless you are in an industrial area that has excellent benefit programs for workers, or you have a thriving, established practice, with many active patients of record, you may not need to worry much about these plans. At least for now! Until your patients move or change jobs. America is a society on the move. Our population shifts constantly and dental offices must always welcome new patients to replace those that move or leave the office. New patients are not educated about their insurance programs and will usually choose the cost-saving alternative plans. If you think that you can hide from these programs and be profitable, you are battling great odds. Also, realize that most practices lose about 20% of their patient base each year. So, you constantly have to bring in new patients to replace those lost.

People are signing up for managed care plans at alarming rates, currently. Some "experts" tell us that we should not worry about this fact because only 50% of the people in our country have dental insurance. I wonder if any of these gurus ever thought what type of patients we get from the other 50%? In my opinion, I cannot count on this segment of the population. Furthermore, the fact is that

80% of the population is middle class or below.

This large segment of population does not want to spend more than a few hundred dollars on their dental care. The 50% segment that does not have dental insurance includes many people who have no employment and not much discretionary income that they are going to spend at your office. I don't see too many un-insured patients waiting to beat a path to my door to spend $2000 on a root canal, core, and crown for one tooth.

The remaining upper segment of the population (20%) is too small to pursue. To try and chase after the 20% of the population that is above middle class is sort of ludicrous. There are another

200,000 dentists trying to do the same thing. And for the most part, this 20% does not necessarily care to spend money on their oral health. They are usually caught up in 80 hour work weeks and business meetings. Don't go chasing pink elephants or black swans. Attempt to serve mainstream America and schedule your career around serving your average American.

Once our country sees a shortage of dentists, instead of a lack of patient pools, then you can stop worrying about managed care. In the meantime, you should realize that you can still perform quality dental care and gain experience treating this patient pool. Yes, you can also earn a comfortable living, as long as you control your schedule. <u>If your chairs are empty you must fill them</u>, in order to be busy performing dentistry 40 hours per week. Accept all types of insurance and use these patients to improve your skills. The more you perform the faster you become. The quicker you begin to complete procedures the more profitable you become. Managed care programs can help you pay your bills, improve your skills, and market your practice. **If you can't beat them, join them. In the meantime, remember that in order to develop your skills you must**

Diagnose, Perform, Repeat!!! The 3 Keys To Success.

I have a colleague who charges approximately twice the usual and customary fee for all of his procedures. He has every diploma and award possible. He is an accredited member of every society out there. He works three days per week and sees approximately three or four patients per day. He is never in a hurry and I have never seen him in distress. The main problem that I have seen with his schedule is that he is not producing. His case acceptance is low because most of his patients seek more affordable care elsewhere. He does some full mouth reconstruction, now and then, but for the most part he is busy polishing his diplomas. While I am busy **doing** four crowns at $1000 he is busy trying to **sell** one crown at $2000. Guess who ends up further ahead financially?

Basic rule: try to make your dental services more affordable to larger segments of the population and work a schedule that allows you to do more dentistry for more people.

This does not mean that you have to diminish quality, or provide poor workmanship. On the contrary, the more you perform, the better you become clinically, and the faster you can do the work. Make yourself available to more patients. Work more, work harder, work more efficiently. Make yourself marketable to more patients and let them spread the word about you. Later on in your career you can consider limiting your patient pool.

Consumers spend more money on gambling, haircare, and tobacco than they do on their dental care. Can you see where people's priorities are? People would rather avoid the dentist than pick up the telephone and make an appointment. <u>Dental needs are way down on people's list of things to purchase.</u> You can set high standards for yourself and your practice, but if you want to serve only the upper echelon of our society, you have to take a serious look in the mirror and ask yourself whether you are better than 99% of the other dentists in your area. Along with this, you must also have some financial backing to be able to open up a state of the art facility and market yourself to that segment of the population. You may just find yourself chasing your tail for too long.

Although I predict that the profession has a bright future, you should not try to fight Goliath. <u>One of the top five insurance carriers has nine times more financial revenue than the entire combined annual US expenditure for dental care and dental products.</u> Prepare and educate yourself. In time, if you decide to limit your patient pool, even the patients on low-fee programs will seek your care and expertise and be willing to cover their own expenses. Patients will follow a caring dentist that has great abilities and excellent human relations skills. And they will be more than happy to pay for their services. But it takes time to build this reputation and trust. And it takes repetition to gain experience and efficiency.

Therefore, you must make yourself available to "Mainstream America" during the early stage of your career.

Dental school taught you the basics. The instructors taught you how to do things the right way in order to avoid re-makes and potential legal problems. This education was a great basis for your future, but it also bred slowness. <u>To be financially and professionally successful you must learn to improve your clinical speed, without sacrificing quality.</u> No matter what type of dentistry you want to practice, you must have a schedule that allows you to do your work at a pace that lets you improve and complete the work to your standards. Quality work can be completed quickly with the proper skills and practice. Lousy work can also be completed quickly with poor skills and improper practice!

One final concept that I want you to think about. With the coming of managed care, patient pools are shrinking. The high-volume practices keep getting bigger while the middle-of-the-road practices keep losing patients. Quality practices continue on the same road to success. Once you have attained excellent communication and clinical skills you do not have to succumb to PPOs and their cousins. Managed care practices will keep growing, while the average, middle of the road offices will slowly disappear. There is going to be an extreme gap in the dental profession. You have to decide which end of the rope you are going to grab. The quality practices will continue to thrive. The large volume practices will flourish. It is the ones on the fence that will have problems. How you practice dentistry your first five years out of dental school will surely dictate where you will be for the rest of your career. Do everything possible to work the way you would like to work and develop the skills that you need to reach your goals. If you find yourself in a situation where you are being told how to do dentistry stand up to your beliefs and work at the pace that you want to work at. Do not give up your principles. If you like fast-paced dental care, then work hard at being quick and efficient without sacrificing your quality standards. Do what you enjoy doing. <u>Do what you believe in! Just don't find yourself sitting on the fence.</u>

Again: Try to make your dental services more affordable to larger segments of the population and work a schedule that allows you to do your type of dentistry for more people.

MAKE IT HAPPEN

BE GOOD TO YOURSELF

BELIEVE IN YOURSELF

CHANGE WHAT YOU WANT TO CHANGE

MANAGE PRESSURE

INSPIRE YOURSELF

OVERCOME LAZINESS WITH GOALS

WHAT YOUR MIND CAN CONCEIVE, YOU CAN ACHIEVE

THE PAST DOES NOT EQUAL THE FUTURE

HAVE BELIEFS

NEVER BE JEALOUS OR RESENTFUL

DON'T WORRY...BE HAPPY

CHAPTER 6
BURN-OUT AND STRESS

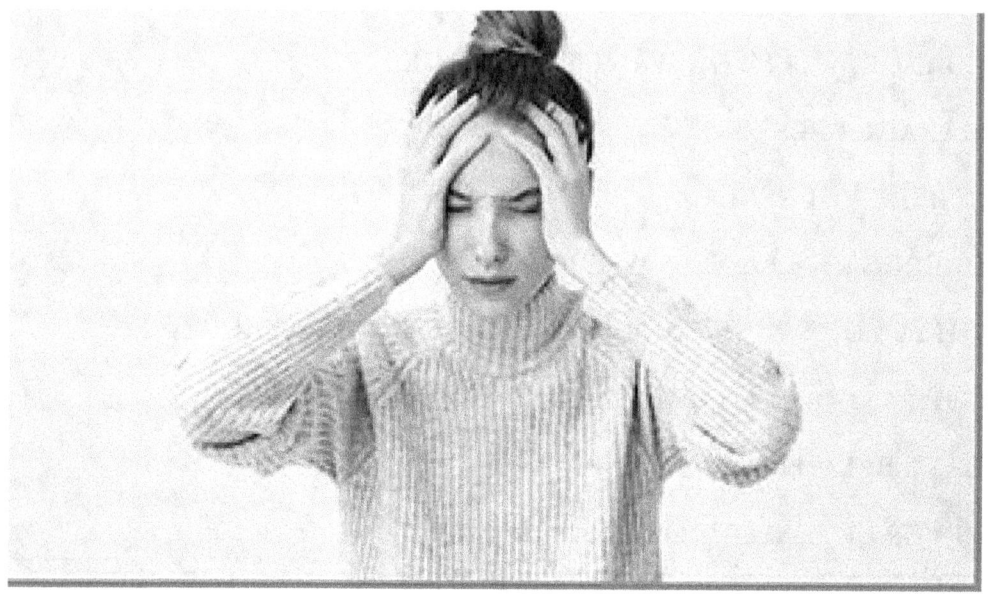

Before you took your first step, you crawled. After that, you were even able to run. The same is true in your professional development. Unfortunately, when you come to the jogging stage, you must learn to slow and balance your stride, before you get too tired. Stress, and even burn-out, are realistic obstacles in dentistry. For this reason, I decided to place this chapter at the beginning of this book. The reader must understand the cumulative effects of stress and learn to balance the daily demands of their dental and personal lives.

A mentor of mine told me that my net profit and professional success will be equivalent to the happiness of the choice that I made to become a dentist. I guess he also meant that this joy must continue indefinitely into my career, otherwise I would stagnate my growth and prosperity. To be happy practicing dentistry you must be happy in your personal life, because it is impossible to be a happy person and a miserable dentist, or vice versa. An unbalance leads to misery and stress.

All people seek food, shelter, money, dignity, and joy (happiness). At the same time all of us try to avoid PAIN.

The pathways that each of us chooses to take will allow us to develop the lifestyle that we desire. Joy can be the result of going down the right track. It may come in the form of socializing, helping people, making money, skiing, playing tennis, diving, etc. In the dental context, joy must come from helping people. It must also be found in the satisfaction of the work that we do, as well as the perception and the frame of mind that we have when we perform the labors of our work. The actions and reactions that we choose will determine how much joy we will have in our lives and how much pain we will avoid. All of us will attempt to avoid certain events, places, people, objects, etc. in order to **avoid PAIN**. It is this negative reaction that leads to much misery, self-doubt, and self-sabotage in our lives. Next time you think about avoiding a difficult patient or a difficult procedure think about why you follow such action. Most likely, it is to avoid a certain amount of pain while trying to focus on another action that will bring you less pain and more joy.

Why did you become a dentist? If you cannot answer this question you may be predisposed to a lot of self-doubt and possibly - stress. Before you read any further, sit down and write your "mission statement." State exactly what you would like to accomplish in your career and why you chose to become a dentist. You can write something as simple as: *"To provide patients with quality dental care in a warm, friendly, professional, and empathetic way. To help relieve pain, improve smiles, enable people to talk and chew, and make a positive improvement in the lives of my patients."* Define your purpose, write it down, and follow it throughout your career. Without a purpose you cannot achieve happiness and joy. You can, however, obtain pain and sorrow. If you mission statement says *"To make lots of money,"* stop reading and send me back this book.

Dentistry is often an overworked profession that is grossly underpaid, and sometimes " joy-less." Many colleagues complain about their hours, the physical demands, the staff, the procedures, the patients, the IRS, etc. These complaints usually multiply as the years go by. The cumulative effects of the daily grind take their toll on many practitioners. This does NOT have to happen to you!

If you learn to follow a fraction of the principles and ideas of this book your career will flower and your life will be happier. Do not listen to the complainers and the cry-babies. Learn to follow the leaders. Stay away from the belief that the grass is always greener on the other side. **Nobody has a perfect job**. Physicians complain of HMOs, firefighters talk about " hitting the wall," golf instructors refuse to play the game, and the list goes on and on. No job, no profession, is perfect or peachy, all of the time. The grass is usually greener in your yard! There are highs, there are lows, and there are plateaus. It is the individual who learns to walk through the valleys that ultimately gets to the top.

You are privileged to be a dentist! And with the guidance of this book you can become one of the happy few. Of course it is challenging to be a dentist. You work in a limited environment and you perform a highly technical job. Besides the physical and mental challenge of the clinical work you must also deal with all of the other facets of the business problems, as well as your personal obstacles. As a dentist you have to be a doctor, technician, employer, human resource director, financial consultant, psychologist, repairman, pseudo-anesthetist, pharmacist, surgeon, pathologist, complaint department, etc. The dental profession challenges you in many ways. You must learn to deal with all of these demands and challenges in a positive manner.

Stress deserves your daily attention, because it is a part of being a dentist. It is also the part of your life that will prevent you from obtaining joy and happiness. Young practitioners have a lot of energy and enthusiasm. As the years go by, the accumulation of daily stress can lead to eventual burn-out (a condition where your physical, emotional, and behavioral states become impaired). You must learn to cope with the daily set-backs, in order to prevent your candle from extinguishing. Of course, you must learn to avoid burning your candle at both ends.

Stress is defined as " the nonspecific (physical, emotional, or behavioral) response of the body to any demand." It is the response to the demand that dictates how your body reacts. Some people never have stress because nothing in the world bothers them. Others reach the burn-out stage and even a traffic jam is a major catastrophe in their daily routine. Avoiding the PAIN of any situation can either be accomplished through positive and affirmative actions or through negative and self-defeating ways. The former leads to a fulfilling lifestyle while the latter accomplishes STRESS.

STRESS LEADS TO PAIN AND VICE VERSA!

ARE YOU GETTING STRESSED?

To self-diagnose the possibility of too much stress in your life consider whether **APATHY** is becoming your worst characteristic. If you are normally an enthusiastic and energetic person that is becoming lethargic and lackadaisical, then there are too many things in your life nagging at you.

I speak to many dental office staff members that complain of their boss throwing instruments and temper tantrums. These are usually the most common manifestations of stress. Others may include loss of appetite, fatigue, feelings of hopelessness, and general irritability. The only way to combat these states is to eliminate your perception of the demands and causative factors, one at a time, while developing a positive frame of mind. Occupational burnout is the root cause of many illnesses and destructive behaviors. It occurs slowly and progressively. The more preventative measures you take to negate the effects of stress, the less likely you are to reach this final stage.

The human body confronts demands through the old, familiar Flight-Fight Response (oh no, Physiology 101). This reaction mechanism functions properly as long as it is not depleted and exhausted. The body adapts and resists, but only to a certain point. Once your energy is zapped, illness sets in. You can try to avoid or minimize the amount of stress experiences, however in today's fast paced lifestyle this is wishful thinking. There are too many demands and events that you have to encounter.

In order to help combat the effects of stress you must understand that stress denotes a response to an initiating demand. This response can be increased heart rate, anger, sadness, guilt, etc. - the opposites of joy. It is not the demand that causes the response, but the meaning that we assign to this stressor, that determines whether or not our Flight-Fight mechanism will be activated, or ultimately depleted. **It is our frame of mind that will channel the effects of the demand.** Each individual has the power to cause or avoid stress. How can this be done when so many things are nagging at you everyday?

Suggestion #1:

Think about the positives of every demand. Rethink negativity!!! Your perception of the potential stress causing event is the deciding factor between normality and stress. Remember, 99.99% of the things in your life are NOT life and death. And, behind every dark cloud is a silver lining. Memorize the following phrase: " Everything that happens, happens for the best!" Most negative events usually lead to something positive once you decide to take the bulls by the horn. Do not be afraid and eliminate the word FEAR from you vocabulary. Substitute the following acronym: **F**alse **E**vidence **A**ppearing **R**eal.

Suggestion #2:

Become pro-active and learn to take control of the negative events in your life. As a dentist, clinical drawbacks are the main stressors of your life. Accept the fact that you are not perfect, and constantly strive to improve your clinical skills. Do not believe that you can perform perfect clinical dentistry. It is not possible, because you are human. Dentistry is an imperfect science. That is the reason we call it the " practice of dentistry." You must realize the realities of the procedures and strive to become the best you can be. Peer contact and continuing education are the keys to improvement. You are working with many different materials and procedures. You must learn how to use the best materials, in order to perform the most proficient procedures. Be pro-active and plan to decrease the number of clinical shortcomings that you may encounter. Master your techniques and improve your knowledge of dental materials. At the same time you must also guard against becoming bored from the repetitious nature of the work. The anxiety that young dentists feel when performing new procedures is slowly replaced by boredom, once that operation is mastered. This monotony becomes another stress factor. Change your routines, upgrade your materials, and alter the way you do things. Change is mandatory to the maintenance of excitement and enthusiasm.

Suggestion #3:

Keep your head high and respect yourself. Dentists are notorious for being known as professionals with low self-esteem. This is usually caused by our patients. We provide them with the best possible care, yet they usually only care about money, fear, and time off from work. Patients usually do not appreciate the effort that we put forth in providing them with the quality of the actual clinical work. You may feel unappreciated a lot more than you may hear words of gratitude. For this reason, you must truly enjoy what you do and you must be enthusiastic about your work. Without true respect for your profession, and without enthusiasm, you will never be able to motivate your patients. Of course, the result will be decreased case acceptance and decreased finances. Never compromise the quality of your dental work because not all of your patients know how to appreciate it. Find gratitude in your abilities. Remember that patients come to you with a problem. Never make that problem your problem. It is always their problem, you are just there to see if you can help with their problem.

Suggestion #4:

Don't worry too much about money at the beginning of your career. Finances are major concerns to most dentists. As a young practitioner you should worry more about improving your personal and clinical skills than attempting to net a quarter of a million dollars. You cannot earn a six-digit income the first five years out of dental school. Your clinical skills are not developed enough. After five years, you should begin to concentrate more on your income, however be careful not to get caught up into the wrong mentality. There are many practice experts speaking at seminars about how they make millions of dollars and retire before they're 50. Before you get caught up in this type of thinking you must realize that a lot of these " full-of-hot-air" speakers are nothing more than city-hopping, seminar speaking, clinically inept dentists that make their money by tooting their New Year's Eve horns at you. Disregard any advice you get from speakers that tell you that they " did," " produced," " grossed," or " made," a million dollars in their office. The only true measure of your success is the quality of treatment that you provide to your patients, the "true" income that you can verify on tax returns, and the balance that you make between your personal and professional life. I know many dentists that make $50,000 a year who are ten times happier than practitioners who make $250,000 a year. You must have some reasonable relationship to reality when you decide to dream of big money in your profession. You can earn as much as you want, to some limited extent, but you will always have to sacrifice something else.

Suggestion #5:

Take control of the events around you! Working in a dental office brings many daily worries and obstacles. Besides the operative aspect, you encounter employee problems, patient complaints, equipment failure, financial set-backs, legal hassles, and a variety of other demands. You must learn to cope with many of these problems through positive adaptation, as well as fore-thought and planning. Most of these drawbacks are usually not deleterious, but often learning experiences that help teach you how to overcome them at a later date. That which doesn't kill, teaches. You have to learn how to control yourself, and your environment, through positive thinking and fore-planning. You have the potential to control the nature and the pace of your work. You also have the ability to control all other aspects of your life. Remember: it is your interpretation of the stressor that causes stress!!! If you cannot learn to control your environment, and the meanings that you assign to certain events, you will have a lot of stress in your life.

Suggestion #6:

Invest time and effort in maintaining a healthy body and an open mind. In order to become successful you cannot blame other things or other people for your problems. You have to gain control of your life through affirmative thinking. This is only possible if you have a healthy mind in a healthy body.

You must care for your body. Invest time and effort into maintaining a healthy body and an open mind. In order to become successful you cannot blame other things or other people for your problems. You have to gain control of your life through affirmative thinking and healthy lifestyle choices. This is only possible if you have a healthy mind in a healthy body.

You must participate in a physical fitness program for your body. This program must include an adequate diet plan. Educate yourself on health,

As humans we constantly seek to gain pleasure and avoid pain. It is part of our basic survival. We all want to feel better, look better, and function at a high capacity....devoid of pain and sickness. This allows us the opportunity to gain pleasure. We see people around us who seem to have boundless energy, function at high performance levels, and have enthusiastic attitudes. We may wonder how one human can be so healthy while another is always suffering from some sort of ailment. More often than not those of us who live below optimal health are often lacking some basic knowledge or insight.

Better health comes from some very simple basic principles. Can our basic necessities be aiding OR causing some of our health ailments, including headaches and migraines?

Our survival depends on 3 basics:
1. AIR
2. WATER
3. FOOD

Clothing and shelter comes next but we are not in shortage of these. Without these basics we cannot survive. But what is today's environment doing to our health? Let's look at these from some simple perspectives.

First, the QUALITY OF AIR continues to be ruined by a very toxic world that we all live in. Pollution, chemicals, auto emissions, ozone depletion, cellular/wireless waves, and electronic transmissions all add to the depletion of oxygen and decrease the quality of the air that we breathe. Although you cannot hide from this you can take some countermeasures to improve the quality of the AIR that you breathe.

1. Use a high quality room air filter/ozonator in your bedroom to clean your air.
2. Keep your windows closed at night
3. Change your furnace filter at least every other month
4. Add healthy plants like Aloe Vera or Lavender in your bedroom
5. Turn off or put the cell phones in another room, away from your bedroom
6. Use organic cleaning products to clean your home
7. Don't leave your TVs or electronics on when you sleep
8. Adults require 7 hours or more of "good sleep" each night for optimal health. Sleeping less than 7 hours or achieving "poor sleep" can be detrimental to your well-being and lead to: headaches, heart problems, depression, obesity, high blood pressure, low metabolism, and even strokes. 30% of the population reports being sleep deficient. If you are depriving

yourself of sleep make the change now to prevent health issues later. If you are getting at least 7 hours of sleep and you still feel tired, with low energy levels, then consider that the quality of your rest may be affected by structural or digestive problems. If you have large tonsils, obstructive nasal passage (thin nose or can't easily breathe through your nose), or sinus issues, you may be struggling to breathe at night. Quality sleep requires proper oxygenation! Get a sleep study

9. Use Breathe Right Nasal strips or Nasal Cones to open your nasal passages. Your sinuses produce nitric oxide which is one of the most important elements that your body uses for metabolism, fighting infections, and keeping you healthy. If you struggle to breathe through your nose (you are a mouth breather) then you will not get any nitric oxide. This can lead to many health ailments including frequent colds and flus.
10. Do breathing exercises if you don't frequent the gym often. Deep breath in, count to 10, exhale! Repeat this at least 10 times every hour. The deeper the breath, the better. It helps to expand lung volume and oxygenation.
11. Buy a good mattress. No matress under $1500 will provide proper support for your spine.

Second, the quality of our WATER has also been ruined by many factors. Tap water is full of chemicals and pollutants. Most water filters can provide enough efficiency to give you clean water to drink. Even a $30 filter is good enough. Bottled water is full of phenols and cancer causing chemicals. **Stay away from bottled water!** Distilled water is pure water and the healthiest hydration for your body. You can buy your own distilling unit as you should never drink water from plastic containers. Also, you cannot drink distilled water solely. Tap water that is filtered still provides the electrolytes that your body needs, but a few cups of distilled water each day is great at removing toxins from your digestive system.

Third:
FOOD AND NUTRITIONAL GUIDELINES FOR A HEALTHY BODY AND...

Many of us would like to have a healthier body and function at a higher capacity, free of ailments, free of pain, free of disease. Unfortunately, this is not always possible. If you want to take the next step towards more optimal health you must begin by making some lifestyle changes. These changes include diet and attitude awareness. This can be like pulling teeth, no pun intended. Not many of us can claim to embody only healthy habits. Habits come from a "comfort zone" of the brain that doesn't concern itself much with value judgments. We know that donuts and candy are bad but they make us feel good so we eat them anyways. Many habits are thus born out of the desire to gain pleasure. The downside of this is that many of these habits often lead to poor health. Yet we hold onto these habits because change itself is stressful.

It has often been said that people will not change until the stress of change is exceeded by the stress of staying the same. A heart attack is a classic example of a person who will trade pizza and burgers for salads, in most cases. However, the "old ways" are a powerful element to be reckoned with. Even after lifestyle changes are made the old ways can prevail.

Do what you've always done, and you'll get what you've always gotten! From a practical perspective, don't waste money on any health improvement programs until you are ready to make a change. It is common for illnesses to recur repeatedly when the desire to "feel healthy" is stronger than the actual willingness and act of doing something about it. Changes that must be made can require a lot of energy and strong-will. We are always looking for the new diet formula, a magic pill in a bottle, or some new drug to make it easy. It does not work that way. Never has, never will.

Recovery from any health conditions means giving the body sufficient time and resources to heal itself. Every message from the heart, mind and soul translates as instructions to the physical body. When people come to realize how dutifully compliant their bodies really are, they may temper their thoughts with more respect. It does not happen overnight. Time is needed. Our general rule of thumb is that: one month of recovery is needed for every year of chronic illness! So, if you are ready for a change: follow these guidelines!

The typical American diet can cause injury and stress to your body, while blocking your body's healing processes. Choosing to upgrade to a healthy diet is one of the most life enhancing decisions you can make. A healthy diet can prevent and reverse illness. Diet changes must be made gradually, yet with ruthless energy and determination. What you eat has a significant effect on your energy levels, your overall health, and your ability to heal. The American diet has become overly convenient. We fill our bodies with choices of food that are quick to prepare or easy to "grab and eat". This can leave us devoid of proper nutrition and balance, as many of these foods lack proper nutrients. We then turn to coffee, vitamins, herbs, and other products hoping that they will make up for our poor choices. Unfortunately, even these can make things worse as the body normally cannot process them efficiently.

Health begins with your digestive system. Besides emotional problems, most illnesses start and end with your gut.

Think of your digestive system as a highway. Cars enter and exit the highway at numerous on/off ramps. These ramps are analogous to your organs. The pancreas, liver, and gallbladder are like entry ramps while the lungs, kidneys, and rectum are like exit ramps. Consider what happens when a crash occurs on the highway and causes a large backup. No cars can enter and few can exit the highway. It is the same thing with your digestive system. Give it chemicals and non-nutritive foods and you have a vehicle crash. The organs get stuck and they stop functioning normally. The only way to start your way to a healthy body is to clean out the crash and get the highway and ramps working again. Turning to vitamins and other promoted fads is usually a waste of money and time. These end up being similar to more vehicles trying to enter the congested highway. They just add more to the problem.

If you have low energy, tire easily, are prone to flus, colds, or other ailments you most likely have a car crash in your digestive system. **The best way to start a nutritional and body healing program is with DIGESTIVE detoxification. This is also called DIGESTIVE CLEANSING.**

This requires your determination to clean your digestive system which in turn will detoxify and

cleanse your entire body. To keep things simple you must remember that you have to "make up" for years of filling your body with chemicals and junk that your body does not need. Order the following product to start the process: https://www.renewlife.com/total-body-cleanse.html
After the 14 day cleanse, start to implement the following habits:

1. Drink 1 cup Prune Juice or Unfiltered Apple Juice with 1 tsp of Psyllium husk every evening

2. **Drink 1 cup freshly juiced Celery juice every morning when you wake up**

3. During the day eat at least 1 cup of organic fruits daily: papayas, berries, mango, watermelon, grapefruit, apricots, apples, figs, and dates.

4. During the day eat at least 2 cups of romaine lettuce, squash, asparagus, kale, spinach. Flavor them with olive oil, peppermint, and sea salt (this being the most important.)

5. Drink at least 1 cup of **Lemon Balm** or Licorice Tea or Red Clover Tea each day (put 1 tsp of **colloidal silver** in any of the teas if you are omitting below Morning Drink)

In about 5 weeks of starting the Detox program YOU WILL START TO SEE HUGE BENEFITS!

You must also make one basic change: CUT OUT THE SUGAR AND THE JUNK! Read the labels of your foods and start avoiding anything that has added sugar or high fructose corn syrup. Splenda and Nutrasweet and all artificial sweeteners are considered sugars in this program.
If you do NOT change any bad diet habits then do not waste your time with these instructions.

Continuing to eat junk food, dairy, white breads, burgers, wheat, soy, corn, canola oil, processed sugar, eggs, pork, farmed fish, gluten, MSG, natural flavors, artificial sweeteners, L-carnitine, whey, whey protein, BREADS, white rice, chips, popcorn, COOKIES, and crackers ...would be analogous to trying to shovel your driveway in the middle of a heavy snowfall.

You must also realize the importance of bacteria in your diet. The human body needs bacteria to survive and live. There are good bacteria (acidophilus, lactobacillus, etc) and then there are bad bugs. The good bugs will be destroyed by antibiotics, sugars, and preservatives. The bad bacteria will be fed by these. So, if you have ever taken antibiotics, or if you like sweets, you have a 100% chance that most of the good bacteria in your body have been destroyed and you have an overgrowth of bad bugs which cause you to have hunger cravings and excess fat storage. Furthermore, you will have an overgrowth of Yeasts, fungus, and molds which are great at sending signals to your brain to make you eat more sugars. One of the bacteria that causes sugar craving signals to your brain is called *methanobrevibacter smithii* and this is one bacteria that loves Splenda and enjoys making you hungry for more.

Ghrelin is called the "hunger hormone", also known as lenomorelin (INN). It is a peptide hormone produced by ghrelinergic cells in the gastrointestinal tract which functions as a neuropeptide in the central nervous system. Besides regulating appetite, ***ghrelin*** also plays a significant role in making us seek and hoard food. When bad bacteria take over your body, the Ghrelin is increased in activity by these bugs. These bad bugs also shield themselves in your body by creating mucus coatings in your GI. These mucus coatings are very hard to eliminate and some people may need more aggressive methods of cleaning the system…above and beyond these instructions.

The only way to increase the level of good bacteria in your body, and thereby lower the level of bad bacteria, is to follow good diet habits and cut out the sugars.

Before you begin with a new eating plan, please realize that the food supply in our country is produced with high levels of toxins and **you MUST AVOID the following**:

1. **MSG, nitrates, nitrites, sulfites preservatives, colorings, carrageenan, BHA, BHT**: all cancer causing chemicals added to keep foods on the shelves longer! If you eat foods out of boxes with long expiration dates, you are filling your body with chemicals.

2. **Sweeteners, such as Splenda, Nutrasweet, Equal**: all cancer producing chemicals that have no nutritional value and break down proper body functions by increasing bad bacteria. Avoid diet products that contain these sweeteners (Diet Coke, Diet Pepsi, diet-most-everything!) Switch to Stevia or use small amounts of honey.

3. **Hydrogenated oils**: evils that are added to foods to make them taste better. Margarine and shortening are made from these and are to be eliminated. Restaurant food is full of these oils so learn to prepare your own meals. Restaurants are unhealthy. You must also avoid frying your foods! Learn to broil, boil, bake, and pressure cook instead. Choose Olive Oil for your cooking

4. **Spices and natural flavorings**: when you see these words on food labels realize that these have nothing to do with any natural products such as pepper, salt, or paprika. They are FDA approved labeling for chemicals being added to foods by manufacturers in order to increase your appetite and get you addicted to the company's particular brand of food.

5. **Pesticides and herbicides**: although helpful in preventing food-borne illnesses they are toxins! Organic foods do not have these chemicals!

6. **High fructose corn syrup**: the most common additive to foods, designed to sweeten your food and get you "hooked" to the taste of the product. It will slowly destroy your pancreas and entire health! This product alone is responsible for many of our ailments. They have tried to relabel it with other names but don't be fooled. Read the labels and see how many grams of sugar each serving has (for example a serving may be one ounce and it can contain 24 g of sugar; eat a few bites and you have consumed 100 g of sugar!). Buy Stevia or organic cane sugar instead of regular sugar for your cooking needs.

7. All Breads (**GRAINS**) are full of sugar and gluten and lectin. Cut out all grains (even if it says whole grain or whole wheat or natural grain, etc.) Look for Ezekiel bread instead as the lesser of evils.

8. **Pastas** (grains) are full of sugar. Try to limit them or buy the Spinach Pasta.

9. **Soy and Milk**

10. **Beans and Tomatoes.** You can peel tomatoes and eat the pulp as an alternative if you really like tomatoes, but avoid the skin. Beans and tomatoes are full of lectins which increase your appetite.

11. **Coffee, Alcohol, and Pork.** These are the 3 Horsemen! Coffee can have mold, alcohol will destroy your liver and increase fungi, while pork is full of toxins.

12. **Smoking**

13. **Cashews and Peanuts.** Stick with Walnuts and Pistachios and limited Almonds.

Please realize that in order to start your health program you must take some initiative and keep things as simple as possible. First, read the labels of the food in your cupboard and refrigerator. Throw out anything that has any of the above compounds. Second, shop for organic products. Even local grocery stores are adding many organic products to their shelves. Focus on finding organic food.

Next, follow some simple rules:

1. **Again: Drink plenty of Filtered Water**: at least half an ounce of water for every pound you weigh, daily! Do NOT ever drink bottled water or straight tap water.

2. **Eat lots of RAW (uncooked) Organic Vegetables**: broccoli, green/red peppers, cucumbers, carrots, squash, tomatoes, avocados, spinach, and other regional greens. Eat as many raw or lightly steamed vegetables and fresh salads as you can digest. Season them with sea salt, extra virgin olive oil, apple cider vinegar, Garlic, ginger, cayenne pepper, chili peppers, and onions. The key is RAW or slightly steamed. If you cook vegetables you lose their enzyme ability. Enzymes are needed for the digestive process to help the pancreas and gall bladder.

3. **Eat the right amount of Proteins:** the best sources are turkey (contains L-tryptophan, a serotonin producing amino acid which helps to stabilize headaches), wild-caught fish (halibut, mackerel, salmon), lamb, cow, and chicken. Avoid farm-raised salmon, tuna. Excellent organic vegetarian protein sources include free range eggs, tempeh, red lentils, and chickpeas.

4. **Consume Complex Carbohydrates:** for sustained energy, eat complex carbohydrates in the form of legumes, red potatoes, squash, yams, and brown rice. Limit your overall carbohydrate intake to 30 percent or less of the foods you eat at each meal.

5. Again: Purchase a room air **filter/ionizer**. You need CLEAN air/oxygen for your lungs.

6. Consult with your doctor regarding your **Vitamin D** and Calcium and Magnesium levels. Many chronic pain patients experience low Vitamin D, calcium, and magnesium levels. Healing requires the proper amount of these critical nutrients for recovery. Your doctor must draw blood for your basic study and ask the lab for the additional specific test for Vitamin D.

7. Add one **Digestive Enzyme** with every meal. Most grocery and pharmacy stores carry these.

8. Add **Flaxseed, Chia Seeds, and Krill Oil** to the diet. Flaxseeds and Chia Seeds can be put into smoothies or oatmeal while Krill Oil supplements can be taken daily.
9. Eat one **APPLE** per day
10. Eat **Sauerkraut and Pickles**
11. Eat lightly steamed **Asparagus and Cauliflower**
12. Take a B-Complex and additional B12 (under your tongue)
13. Take Magnesium supplements
14. Take Vitamin C

FUNCTION:

As part of Digestion and Food come your jaws and teeth. Obviously as a dentist you know that if you have missing teeth or an abnormal occlusion (bite) you are most likely deficient in proper jaw function. Impaired mouth structure and function can lead to abnormal breathing, digestion, health ailments, and pain. Fix your dentition the same way you would fix your patients'!

Grinding and clenching teeth is an issue that affects over 25% of the population. This can cause an impact on over 45% of your nervous system function. Controlling clenching and bruxing issues is one of the most important treatments that dentists can offer to patients. Wear an NTI or upper discluding orthotic.

AMALGAM FILLINGS AND REMOVAL

Removal of amalgam fillings is toxic to your body. The aerosol vapor released during removal will get ingested into your lungs and fall on your eyes, hair, and skin. Subsequently it will deposit into your organs and tissues. This will cause you a multitude of health problems: itchy skin, nervous system debilitation, endocrine disturbances, tachycardia, emotional instability, headaches, tinnitus, hearing loss, insomnia, breathing problems, allergies, tremors, headaches, fatigue, thyroid swelling, cognitive impairment, etc..

Although the debate on this topic continues please consider why your dental office is mandated by the government to have amalgam separators installed. These devices remove mercury from the evacuation lines. The reason is that the FDA considers the removal of silver (amalgam) fillings to be a toxic procedure as the mercury is released during drilling. Mercury is considered a toxic element by the FDA and it needs to be removed before entering sewer lines or waterways. If silver fillings were safe we would not need amalgam separators to keep the environment safe. In Europe amalgam has been banned for a long time.

Mercury has also been removed from thermometers and even a small spillage in a chemistry lab causes an emergency protocol to be implemented.

As a dentist who removes amalgams you are at high risk. Take precautions to remove amalgams safely:

1. use a rubber dam
2. use an extraoral suction
3. cover yourself with full PPE
4. cover your assistant with full PPE
5. cover your patient with full PPE
6. use a respirator
7. use hair gown
8. use face shield
9. use safety goggle and mask over your patient's ears
10. discard all PPE at end of procedure.

Prevention is the key!

Some additional advice:

11. Exercise a minimum of three times per week, including strengthening your back muscles. Visit a physical therapist, or trainer, for specific advice. Learn to balance your work-out program.
12. Visit a chiropractor on a regular basis!!!
13. Avoid alcohol and tobacco.
14. Enjoy nature.
15. Do Yoga.
16. Have hobbies.
17. Take a week off every 2-3 months.
18. Drink water when tired.
19. Medidate and think with an open mind.

Furthermore, as a dentist you are constantly bombarded with the need to solve problems. Here is a list of the demands and actions that I have personally encountered in the last few weeks (pay attention to some of the management principles):

1. X-Ray unit down... rescheduled one patient because all of the other rooms were full; offered a 10% discount for inconvenience; called repairman; ordered another chair and x-ray (I guess the practice was busier than I realized).
2. Yesterday's root canal patient still having pain...changed ATBs, reduced occlusion, and prescribed more Decadron. Showed extreme empathy!!!
3. Accountant called and declared we needed to amend last year's returns...spend five hours researching income and expense reports.

4. Hygienist decided to move to California...hired new doctor (increased production and new patient flow).
5. Office administrator's car broke down and kids were sick...moved one assistant to front area and increased hours for other assistants.
6. Aluminum siding in front office blown off by high winds...made ten phone calls and finally found a repairman.
7. Estimate for front office remodeling doubled...fired contractor, drew up new plans with different company (received twice the value for half the price).
8. Had a 25% increase in failed appointments...reviewed Call Source tapes and evaluated the staff's telephone etiquette (new training implemented, removed one assistant from duties of scheduling, and shazam).
9. Itero system blew up...called company and got replacement.
10. Recalls down 30%...took out the whip, mailed postcards, emailed promotion ...25 recall phone calls within 5 days.
11. Two deadbeat patients refused to pay their bills threatening to sue for malpractice...informed my lawyer who filed summons and complaint (received money within two days).
12. A rash of smokers would not numb for lower amalgams...prescribed Valium, dispensed Benadryl, and rescheduled (no problem second time around).
13. Three root canals with four, curved canals...increased appointment time (had lots of fun).
14. Periodontal surgery patient not performing hygiene...requested signature for admission of my " inform," sold Sonicare, showed slides of denture patients, scheduled back for two months (gained patient respect, since I show concern, but never scold patients about their hygiene).
15. Patient complained that I gave her a price that was $50 higher than the final fee...accepted adjusted payment, re-studied my fees and treatment plan sheet, re-evaluated my communication process, and re-affirmed front office staff need to finalize price explanations.
16. Porcelain veneer broke during try-in...re-evaluated prep, Patient got free T-shirt and tickets to the movies.
17. PFM #19 did not fit...realized it was an Itero issue. Free ice-cream cone for this patient.
18. Lower Unilateral Partial distorted at final delivery, despite fitting at try-in appointment...called lab, redesigned case (maintained calm with lab person who has a lot more stress than the rest of us do).
19. Patient not pleased with contours of Class IV composite...recontoured and custom shaded (decided to stop doing large composites and treatment plan more porcelains).
20. Two lab deliveries late...rescheduled patients, re-evaluated shipping procedures, scheduling, and job responsibilities (gave patients mugs and T-shirts).
21. PFM crown #30 placed two weeks ago flared up...performed root canal and had happy patient (who was previously instructed as to the possibility).
22. Belligerent patient wanted more narcotics...dismissed from practice (received standing ovation from staff).
23. Allergic to penicillin patient was prescribed Cleocin and had a seizure while driving; paramedics called me upon her request...send patient to hospital for hypersensitivity treatment (immediately reviewed pharmacology of common ATBs). Neurologist called and told me it is very common for patients to develop seizures from medications. Now prescribing only Azithromycin since Clindamycin products getting such bad rap.

24. Old patient showed up with fractured PFM #20 which I had placed two years ago...replaced at half cost, since I already explained the possibility of porcelain breakage on posterior teeth (patient very delighted with the half-cost).
25. Found dental assistant emailing her resumes to department stores...scheduled private meeting to decide what the problem was (employee felt unappreciated and overworked...re-learned lesson about employee needs; all calm now).
26. Four surface, two-week old composite on #10 looked great, but tooth throbbing...finished root canal and received gratitude from patient, who was informed of the depth of decay at previous appointment.
27. Started core/crown procedure on patient who refused other than BW XRs at initial appointment; P.A. of posts revealed improper root canal seal and large apical lucency...performed root canal re-treatment and temporization until healing observed (patient felt like a fool for denying FMX, while I kicked myself in the rear for starting a large procedure without a P.A.- cardinal sin #1).
28. New patient told administrator that her appointment was painful...called patient and re-emphasized our concern (prescribed Valium and suggested NO2 for next appointment; stressed the need for her to feel in control and stop us if she feels discomfort; scheduled an easy procedure on an upper tooth; keep fingers crossed that she returns).
29. Wife complained about golfing all day Sunday...tee-times reduced to 9 holes. No range balls.
30. Parents complained about not visiting...brought over steaks and fish and barbecued (left food bill with dad).
31. Stock broker called with news that two of my stocks went belly-up...researched my portfolio and restructured. Decided money in my business was better than my money on Wall Street.
32. Oral Surgeon called with final diagnosis of swollen submandibular gland (differentially diagnosed as sialolith): Stage II Lymphoma. Send this patient flowers and picked up the Oral Diagnosis book.
33. Patient's husband called and requested to discontinue partial denture treatment due to finances...put case on shelf and advised patient that lab deposit would be forfeited (patient appreciated loss of investment).
34. Patient with pre-determination clause in insurance contract received rejection of 10 amalgams due to our failure to send in pre-determination...allowed a rare payment plan (patient canceled insurance and so did 20 of her co-workers; back at the ranch we reviewed the need to send pre-determinations for all contracts that require it).
35. Emergency root canal patient changed jobs and lost insurance while pulling a Houdini act...wrote off debt after unsuccessfully trying to collect; decided to sue insurance company - no result, yet. Part of doing business.
36. Late afternoon Saturday patient walked in to office with fractured anterior demanding treatment on his 100% coverage plan. Could not confirm insurance coverage...rescheduled for Monday (guess what???...no insurance!!!).
37. New dental assistant stopped coming to work after two days...instructed other employees to start a new search (four qualified applicants in four days).
38. Bruised shins kick-boxing...ordered shin guards and wobbled for a few days.
39. Ran out of air scuba diving...purchased another tank and increased exercise program.
40. New Patient flow down by 25 from our usual 85 per month...new postcards mailed; 20 new patients within 10 days.
41. Lab behind on two bridges...send lab person on vacation (he was hitting the proverbial wall)

42. Received rejection letter from my building insurance company stating that my damaged windows (punks with bi-bi guns) would not be covered in full...canceled four of my policies and received better coverage for less money with another company.
43. Wife complained of lack of attention...scheduled two rummy appointments and two dinner dates; received back massage and clean laundry.
44. Overdenture patient called and complained of loose fit... relined and replaced two male connectors (patient lost weight).
45. Numerous perio patients called and complained of severe sensitivity to cold...evaluated our post-op protocol and found that patients were not being instructed as to the proper use of Fl and sensitive toothpaste.
46. Denture patient complained of loose lowers...for the 135th time, re-explained the problems with lower fits and referred her to surgeon for implants and vestibular extension (patient still did not understand, so I recorded the conversation and emailed it to her to review; instructed staff to tell patient that I moved to Leningrad). Made sure that all fees were collected pre-op!!!
47. Veneer #5 broke at the mesio-distal line angle. Patient was President of the UAW Branch. Repaired with composite at no charge. Received four new patients from the local 192.
48. Four year old went ballistic. Send him to specialist via air mail. Entire family appointed for treatment after seeing what happens in a pedo office, compared to our office.
49. Severe back-pain for two days. Left work early, dashed to the club for intense strengthening exercises and called chiropractor. Took 2 days off and watched Looney Tunes.
50. Lab lost TMJ orthotic. Gave patient $100 credit on account.
51. Tenant not sure about renewing lease...called agent and received 10 interested parties in 2 days (raised rent 25% and got quick decision).
52. Computer down...called support, made light threats, got fixed (never worked better).
53. Collections down 15% for the month...found untracked claims (had eye-eye meeting with insurance coordinator).
54. Four patients switched to managed care plans this week...send letter and magnet (they'll be back!!!)
55. Rash of sensitive posterior composites...decided to use more primer/bond, more irrigation, more Gluma, and check occlusion closer. Also implemented 50:50 solution for all decay removal.
56. Broken new lower denture...decided to add metal reinforcement for all lower dentures in the lingual anterior area.
57. Three 2-hour appointments canceled at the last minute. Implemented new policy of requiring down-payments for long procedure appointments. Evaluated communication process and decided that patients were just boneheads.

The list goes on and on. The common denominator is that <u>all stressful events are learning episodes</u> that teach you how to become better and overcome their duplicity in the future. Most of these problems can have a deleterious effect on your life, if you allow them to. It is up to you to chose not to let this happen. Become optimistic, develop a positive frame of mind, and deal with demands in a happy and pro-active manner. It is the only way to diminish the effects of stress and enjoy a happy life. But always remember: if you keep doing the same thing over and over and expecting different results… Make sure you always learn and adapt!

To take control of your life, you must be able to make decisions and take immediate action. Whenever you encounter a difficult situation that can lead to stress and pain, ask yourself:

1. What joy and pleasure will you miss from not taking action?
2. What benefits will you get from taking action and how will it enhance your life, now and later?
3. What will you avoid by taking action and what can happen if you don't take action?
4. If I don't do it, then who will?

All human beings have the ability to change themselves and their destiny. If you ever find yourself in doubt of your future and you feel frustrated by everything around you, then follow this advice:

1. Change your breathing and your posture…breathe deeper and keep your head up high.
2. Smile and make yourself be happy.
3. Indulge in things that inspire you.
4. Change your 'State."
5. See yourself in five years and ask yourself if you like what you see if you don't change your "State."
6. Change your core beliefs. Change from, "I don't see how I can do this," to "I know I can accomplish this."

AVOID:

- ANGER
- WORRYING
- FRUSTRATION
- SELF-PITY
- LONELINESS

BE:

- HAPPY
- INTELLIGENT
- HEALTHY
- HUMOROUS
- OUTGOING

NEVER LIMIT YOURSELF

EACH FAILURE IS ANOTHER LESSON

HAVE VALUES

WHAT IS MOST IMPORTANT IN YOUR LIFE? write it down now:

CHAPTER 7
YOUR GOALS AND PLANS

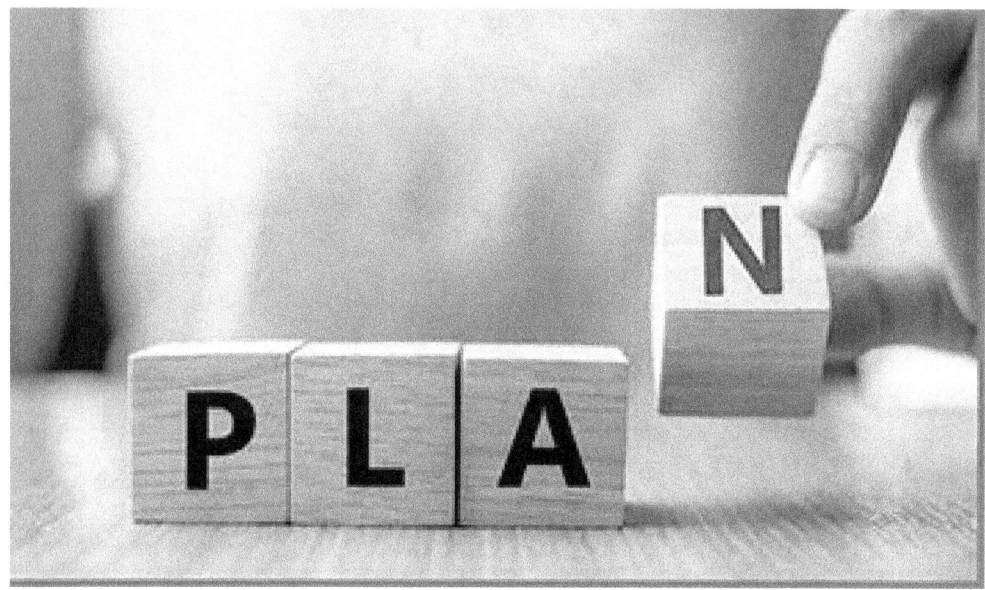

A professional without goals is like a ship without a steer, like a kite without rope. Your future depends on your ability to set goals, priorities, and follow through with determination to achieve those goals. Everyday in dental school you had projects to accomplish and things to get done. These were set goals!!! As you are no longer in dental school, there is nobody to set these goals for you. You're on your own. What you want to achieve in your personal and professional life depends on your ability to set goals. Without setting goals you will be driving through life with blinders on. Once you decide to set your goals clearly your mind will de-fog itself and give you the energy to help you achieve what you want to. It's almost like turning on your rear-windshield de-fogger during a cold winter day.

Without goals, you're stuck in quicksand. Once you know what you want to do, write it down, figure out how to do it, and go for it. The first step is to figure out **what you want to achieve in your life and WHY** you are committed to reaching these goals. It is great to have ambition and motivation to try and achieve certain goals, but this is not enough. You must ask yourself why you want to achieve what you want to accomplish and why it is so important for you to do so. If you cannot answer the WHY part then your goal becomes meaningless and its attainment useless.

On the other side of the coin, you must also ask yourself what will happen if you do not set and reach your goals. What will you think thirty years from now? Will you look back upon your life and consider it a failure? Or will you sit in your rocking chair and remember all of the things that you have accomplished in your life? Your goals must be able to drive you every day and the reasons you give towards attaining them must be strong enough and " real" enough in your mind to help you achieve them.

The first aspect of setting goals is to write down your goals on a piece of paper and keep it for future reference. Daily, you must review your goals and take the necessary steps to achieving those goals. Don't write these down unless you have figured out a way to achieve them You must be sensible and practical. Winning the lottery is not a goal. Learning molar endo and orthodontics next year is a goal.

Before we begin a few exercises you must realize that everything around you once began as a goal. Edison's light bulb was an idea and a goal that took thousands of tries and many years of hard work to accomplish. The chair you're sitting in was once somebody's goal. The car you drive was a goal. The T.V you watch was a goal. Everything around you was once a goal. These things came to be because somebody wanted them realized. Those people set goals to achieve what they dreamt and they accomplished their goals through hard work, determination, and positive frame of mind.

And they all asked themselves one basic question: "Why do I want to do this?"

Ford invented the assembly line because he wanted to put the world on wheels. Edison wanted to light the world. And you will set your goals because you want to achieve them for a specific reason. Obviously your starting point is to ask yourself what you want to achieve and WHY. Without giving yourself logical reasons you will never achieve your goals. Think about the WHY part whenever you set goals.

If you can't answer to yourself why you want to achieve a certain goal you will not have meaning or reason for your goal.

On the last three pages of this chapter you will find some tables that I want you to Xerox. Go copy them now and then come back to reading. Grab the first table, " Personal Goals," and start writing down all of the goals that you would like to set for yourself. Take ten minutes to do this and then stop. Don't break the ten minute rule. Not a minute longer and not a minute shorter. These goals are for the purpose of making you become the person you want to be. They can be such simple things as learning to scuba dive, learning to play a piano, taking karate lessons, reading certain books, losing weight, making certain friends, undertaking different activities, doing so and so with your family, devoting time to charity, etc. Expect the best for yourself without limitations. Write down everything you would like to accomplish in your personal life. Write as many goals as you can, in ten minutes, and give yourself a certain time frame to achieve them. Worry more about thinking of what you want, instead of when you want to accomplish it. You have ten minutes!

When you are finished I want you to pick out THREE of the most important goals and list them on three by five cards, as follows:

GOAL:
WHY I WANT TO ACHIEVE:
TO BE ACHIEVED BY: (date) this time next year
HOW TO ACHIEVE:
OBSTACLES:
REVIEW GOAL EVERY (i.e. month):

These three goals are going to be your main personal goals for the next year. You must achieve them. No excuses. You will keep the other goals listed and you will do this exercise again in 12 months. But for now, you will strive to achieve these three goals that will help you become the person that you want to become, in the next 12 months.

Grab the next piece of paper, entitled " Materialistic Goals," and start writing down as many things as you want to have in your life. Be as modestly greedy as you want to be. List cars, homes, boats, vacation condos, dental practices, and any other materialistic things that you want to have in your life. When your ten minutes are up pick the top THREE and define them.

GOAL:
WHY I WANT TO ACHIEVE:
TO BE ACHIEVED BY: (date) this time next year
HOW TO ACHIEVE:
OBSTACLES:
REVIEW GOAL EVERY (i.e. month):

Obviously you need to be realistic and cerebral about your material desires. On a dentist salary you are not going to buy the Taj Mahal in 12 months. Be realistic, but do not be afraid to set high priorities for yourself. Just try to stay within your capabilities and earning potential. Also, attempt to categorize these goals into five, ten, and twenty year plans.

Last, but not least, grab the last piece of paper entitled " Financial Goals," and do the same thing you did for materialistic goals. It would be helpful for you to read a book on investments before setting these goals. You can set investment goals such as stock and bond purchases or real estate transactions. Try to develop a scheme of financial planning for your future. Again, do this in a one, five, ten, and twenty year outlook. Consult with a financial planner, if you so desire. You have three days to finish this list.

After you finish this exercise your mind will start to wander and you will come up with many other ideas for your existing goals and other goals that you may want to add to the list. Do not let your desires fall by the roadside. Here are a few suggestions that you should follow:

1. Carry pen and paper with you at all times (write down a daily to-do-list, as well as any other ideas you may get).
2. Go to your nearest office supply store and purchase a set of 3x 5 cards. Begin to write down all of your goals, as follows:

GOAL:
WHY I WANT TO ACHIEVE:
TO BE ACHIEVED BY: (date) this time next year or in 5, 10, 20 years
HOW TO ACHIEVE:
OBSTACLES:
REVIEW GOAL EVERY (i.e. month):

Your goals must be in writing. Many of them will be small goals (i.e. learning about new bonding agents or improving your computer knowledge or learning to sky-dive). Goals must be specific and clearly outlined. They must be evaluated and reviewed often. Allow for changes, additions, and deletions to your progression, but do not give up on your goals. All realistic goals can be achieved with the right vision and determination. If you are making life-long goals you must also make short-term goals that help you achieve them. Lifetime goals may be vague and they need to be defined by more specific and action oriented short-term goals. Before you received your dental degree you had to pass hundreds of courses and tests. Your main goal of being a dentist was achieved through numerous short-term actions and achievements.

You must allow for constant outside help and education. Read books, attend seminars, listen to tapes, and seek people that will help you achieve your goals. Eliminate non-productive tasks and duties during your daily activities. Stick to your guns and learn how to use your environment to help you achieve your goals.

The following company has some of the best educational material available to help you understand more about goals and other self-improvement projects.
www.nightingale.com

The dictionary defines a goal as "the end result toward which effort is directed." Your daily activities must be directed towards your goals. Motivation comes from your ability to define the reason for your goals (the WHY) and your determination to achieve them. You must remember to write down your goals. It makes your vision tangible and increases the chances of achievement. It also helps you to visualize your goal and gives you the ability to refer to it for modifications. Writing also provides positive reinforcement and energy.

Don't be afraid to fail. The best ideas in modern history took hundreds of failures before they became advances. You must act despite fear. Courage comes from the ability to make mistakes and take chances. Don't dwell on losses, mistakes, and shortcomings. Lose the perfectionism characteristic that most dentists inherit upon graduation from dental school. You are human and you cannot be perfect. Perfection never meets reality. Goals never achieve without trial and error. Tell yourself constantly "I can," and "I will." You will not stumble upon destiny; it comes as a matter of choice and willingness. When you decide to be successful, you will be.

A few goals that you should work on are as follows:

Goal #1 (Personal):

Develop great communication skills in order to motivate people. Without the ability to express your thoughts, feelings, and knowledge you have no avenue that leads you towards excellent human relations and people skills. Believe it or not, your success depends on your ability to communicate with others. Success is compromised by technical knowledge and human relations skills. The former constitutes about 10% of your success, while the latter compromises at least 90%. During your infant career stage you must absorb the skills to become a great communicator. Mastering the art of effective human relations is just as important as improving your clinical skills.

The business of dentistry is not the business of filling teeth - it is a business of people. This goal will take time and practice.

TO BE ACHIEVED BY: constant improvement for the rest of my life
HOW TO ACHIEVE: read the following books _____
           listen to the following tapes _____
           practice two communication strategies daily
OBSTACLES: myself, busy schedule, boneheads, and morons
REVIEW GOAL EVERY: week

Goal #2 (Personal):

Take care of your body, mind, and soul. Read the previous chapter again. Learn to balance your professional life with the ability to love, play, and believe. Take care of your health by exercising and eating right. Take care of your mind by expanding it with other non-dental related hobbies or interests. Stay in touch with your religious or other spiritual beliefs. This goal must be made on a daily basis.

TO BE ACHIEVED BY: daily
HOW TO ACHIEVE: join exercise program at ___
           read the following books _____
           listen to the following tapes _____
           make time every other day for _____
OBSTACLES: busy schedule, family events, etc...
REVIEW GOAL EVERY: day

Goal #3 (Personal/Materialistic/Financial)

Become the best clinician possible. It will improve your personal life as well as your financial and material goals. Go above and beyond the normal requirements to improve your skills and become a top-notch practitioner. Be careful not to fall into the trap of trying to be perfect. Set multiple goals. For example, you may want to improve your impression technique for crowns:

TO BE ACHIEVED BY: August 16
HOW TO ACHIEVE: take the following course and read the following book ____

OBSTACLES: money, time
REVIEW GOAL: August 17

Remember:
1. Define the goal (WHY!).
2. Figure out how to achieve the goal.
3. Write down the goal.

PERSONAL GOALS

GOAL	TIME FRAME	REASON I WANT TO ACHIEVE
1.		
2.		
3.		
4		
5.		
6.		
7.		
8.		
9.		
10.		
11.		
12.		
13.		

Notes:

MATERIAL GOALS

GOAL	TIME FRAME	REASON I WANT TO ACHIEVE
1.		
2.		
3.		
4		
5.		
6.		
7.		
8.		
9.		
10.		
11.		
12.		
13.		

Notes:

FINANCIAL GOALS

GOAL	TIME FRAME	REASON I WANT TO ACHIEVE
1.		
2.		
3.		
4		
5.		
6.		
7.		
8.		
9.		
10.		
11.		
12.		
13.		

Notes:

You do not have to be Einstein to set and achieve your goals.

GENIUS = 1% INSPIRATION, 99 % PERSPIRATION!

Obstacles are opportunities that need extra energy in order to achieve goals.

Enthusiasm, achievement, and happiness are the result of motivation to succeed.

Success and happiness are achieved when you set goals according to your values.

Motivation requires little energy when you do what you enjoy.

Love what you do! Believe in what you are doing!

If dentistry makes you happy, it becomes easier to set goals and achieve them.

GOALS = SELF-MOTIVATION.

GOALS MAKE YOU REALIZE WHY YOU ARE BUSY.

SUCCESS IS UNATTAINABLE WITHOUT GOALS.

GOALS MUST BE SPECIFIC AND REALISTIC.

POSITIVE MENTAL ATTITUDE IS REQUIRED TO REACH YOUR GOALS.

SUCCESS GOAL + PLAN OF ACTION + DETERMINATION + POSITIVE FRAME OF MIND.

All of the above information will help you get started towards achieving your future, however you must begin by planning your steps to attaining your goals. We have not covered the basics of figuring out how to go about achieving your goals because it is up to you to figure out how to do so. To help you better understand the requirements for establishing your steps you must begin by taking a good look in the mirror. Most dentists are plagued with a personality and demeanor that I can best describe as being gutless, spineless, and wimpy. This type of personality usually leads to self-defeat and an inability to take control of their lives and goals. Your average American dentist is a nerdy wimp who is happy with his garbage man salary and mediocre lifestyle. His goals are usually modest and easily achievable. He usually talks himself out of a better life and a brighter future due to an inner pessimism and defeatist attitude.

(Author's note: The masculine reference to "he," wherever you see it in this book, does not in any way indicate any bias or prejudice on my behalf. If you would - please - regard any reference to "he" as a generalization that encompasses all genders and races of dentists.)

If you have set big goals for yourself and you have finished giving them a timetable then you must hold your head up high and believe that you can achieve anything that you have envisioned. Lose the wimp attitude and walk with pride, on a daily basis. Ask yourself the following, "What will happen if I do not achieve my goals and what will I lose in my life?" Also, change your way of thinking from the old " I have to" to a more optimistic " I want to," or " I desire to," and start believing in yourself and your abilities. Get out of the survival mode and enter the achievement mode!!! You want and desire to do certain things in your life because ___.

All people on this planet do things because they want to avoid pain and gain pleasure. Review your goals and you will realize that they all basically have this common denominator. You want to be a great clinician because you want to avoid the pain of re-doing your work, or possibly being sued. You also want to achieve pleasure by seeing the end-result: quality work. You want to earn more money because you want to gain the pleasure of buying certain things that give you pleasure. You want to improve certain personal attributes because they make you feel better about yourself and you want to gain the pleasure of being known as a great person. You want to set up a retirement account because you want to avoid the pain of being poor when you get older. **Just think about everything that you do and you will realize that you do things in order to avoid pain and gain pleasure.** Use this knowledge to master your emotions and gain the determination to help you achieve your goals.

Do not be afraid to believe in the principle that the body can achieve what the mind can dream of. It is a great " theory," as long as you know your limitations and your abilities. Remember: be realistic, otherwise you will fail and become miserable! If you want to make a million dollars a year as a dentist, figure out a way to do so. It's possible and it is being done by hundreds of successful dentists. However, you should figure out a different way to do so, other than daily bread and butter dentistry. You're not going to make a million smackers doing amalgams. If you want to dunk a basketball and you're only 5 foot 3 inches tall then you better get in the gym five times a week.

I see a lot of dentists attending seminars that will help them become better dentists and achieve successful, quality dental practices. I also see a lot of dentists wanting to become cosmetic dentists. These are great goals to set for yourself as long as you figure out a way to achieve them. For example, if you want to be a cosmetic dentist you must research your patient base, geographic/economic make-up, and your skills. If you want to go to Hollywood and work on movie stars, you have to ask yourself whether you can market yourself and be able to rub noses with the right people, in order to stimulate the appropriate referrals. At the same time, if you want a quality oriented dental practice you must sit down and list all of the different things you must do to get people to realize that you are a quality dentist. You can't just say "I want to be a quality dentist" and work with outdated equipment. You must figure out a way to become that practitioner and let people know, and see, that you are that type of dentist. Every goal must be realistic and every goal requires a plan of action.

Finally, review your goals again:

Short Term (one year or less)
Medium Term (five years or less)
Long Term (five years and more)

Make them realistic! Make them achievable!

GOALS: EFFORT AND COURAGE ARE NOT ENOUGH WITHOUT PURPOSE AND DIRECTION

CHAPTER 8
TO BE OR NOT TO BE

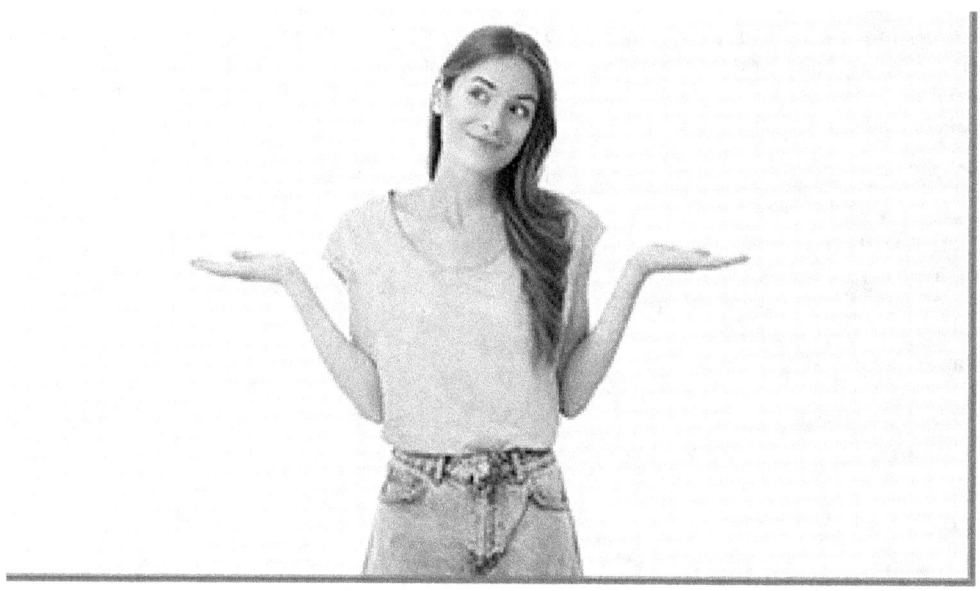

Should you, or should you not open your own dental office? Do you want to be a practice owner? Do you want to buy an existing office or open one up from scratch? Have you thought about this goal? If yes, have you written it down? Whatever your desires may be, my basic suggestion is as follows: do not do so until you have gained enough clinical experience, and business knowledge, to keep your head above water. The easiest gauge of this experience is simple: when you can do a molar root canal, core, and crown in less than 70 minutes you are ready for ownership. I get too many telephone calls from recent graduates who are itching to open up their own office, or buy an existing practice. Today's business climate and managed care environment weeds out the inexperienced and anxious practice owners. The next chapters will give you a little more insight in terms of office management and business protocol, however to keep things simple, I will offer a few words of advice for the anxious practice owner.

Buying an existing dental practice is often the easiest and fastest way to become owner. The drawbacks, however, usually outweigh the benefits. If you decide to buy an existing practice you are also buying that office's headaches, problems, and shortcomings. You may certainly be able to do "The Profit" on this business however that requires a lot of knowledge and experience.

First, you must find a well-managed and established practice. Your local brokers may be helpful. If you want to go this route, your best option is to work as an associate with a "sweat equity buy-in" whereby the owner gives you shares of the business while you work and make money and grow that practice. Determine the value of the business and the terms before you start working there especially since you will most likely help to grow the business and increase revenues and profit.

Some practitioners will list the sale of their offices through state dental association journals. These practices need to be evaluated carefully and with the help of professionals. The most valuable and easiest sale transactions involve the buy-out of practices by the junior associate. If you are lucky to be in this situation you have an inside track.

Once you have found a practice to buy, you must take many different things into consideration. No matter how you found the practice, you must treat the purchase as a business transaction, with absolutely no personal feelings involved. Your accountant and business attorney will be very helpful, in terms of helping you evaluate and appraise the business. Do not attempt to go at it alone!!! If you need more advice, feel free to reach out and contact me for help.

But....Do your homework! Brokers will always embellish the "brochure" and it is up to you to look between the lines and figure out what you are buying.

Take the following things into consideration if you want to buy a practice:

1. How efficient is the staff and will your personalities blend? Evaluate the efficiency and productivity of the employees!
2. What percentage of overhead is being spent on staff cost? Above 25% could indicate inefficiency and other problems!
3. What is the historical turn-over rate of employees, and how often do you expect to be hiring and training new personnel?
4. Is the geographic area conducive to finding new and adequate staff members?
5. Is the office location centrally located and easily visible?
6. Does the office have large signage that is easily visible from the road?
7. What is the layout of the "plant" and can you perform dentistry efficiently with this set-up? Are you limited by the number of ops and can you grow in the future/
8. What is the value of the dental equipment? Ask your local dental supplier to evaluate.
9. What is the value of the dental supplies?
10. What remodeling needs does the office have, and how much will they cost?
11. What type of patients are being treated (cash, PPO, Fee-for-service, etc.)?
12. How many active patients are there (seen within last 12 months)?
13. Is the office computerized? Is the computer up to date and "clean"?
14. What is the basic overhead, based on the last 24 months?
15. What is the P & L for past 3 years
16. How many new patients is the practice seeing per month and is there room to market to new patients? What is the cost to acquire new patients?
17. What are the gross revenues for the last two years and can you expect to service your debt while putting food on the table?
18. Will you be performing the same services as the selling dentist? Very important! If you can provide many of the referred out services you can double a practice within 12 months.

However, if the selling dentist does implants and root canals and ortho and you won't learn to do those, then your business will go bankrupt. Simple as that! Look at what is being done clinically and the best purchase will always be the one where you can expand and not shrink services. GET A FULL BREAKDOWN OF PRODUCTION BY PROCEDURES SUMMARY.

19. Are you as fast and efficient clinically as the last dentist?
20. How many hours did the previous owner work to generate his practice income?
21. What is the collection rate and how many problem accounts are there?
22. What is the patient education and communication process like?
23. Do you really want to rely upon your " sixth sense" or " gut feeling"?...there is only one type of matter found in your intestines!
24. Can you evaluate the quality of the dental work being performed in this office? Will you spend a lot of your time fixing somebody else's work? Look at BWs of seated crowns and Pas of root canal fills and you will know quickly.
25. What is the quality of the current marketing avenues and how does the website look?
26. What are the current patient reviews about the office?
27. What are the prior 3 years collection figures and are the trends up or down?
28. Does Hygiene produce at least 25% of the revenue? If less than 25%, you may need to hire new hygienists. If Hygiene Department produces more than 25% of the revenue, it means the selling dentist is lazy and you can easily improve doctor production.
29. What is the A/R? Anything above 125% of monthly collections indicates a need to retrain personnel.
30. How about the accounts payables? Are vendors trying to collect their money?
31. Are there liens or heavy debt on the practice or building?
32. Does previous doctor have any litigation in past 5 years?
33. Are the fees lower than UCR fees? Look at ADA fees by geographic area to compare. A simple 10% fee hike can potentially put 100k in your pocket.

Many, many other questions and topics need to be addressed if you decide to purchase an office. Obviously, financing is going to be the main obstacle facing the transaction. If the owner is going to provide you with a reasonably termed land contract (the owner sells the practice to you and also becomes the lender) your problems are solved. These sales are the most common way of becoming a practice owner, especially in a "sweat" position. They are an easy way of transitioning a young dentist into the position of owner. Keep the interest rate at the prime and remember that the owner is more anxious than you to finalize the deal. **However, if you have to seek bank financing do not be afraid as banks currently love to give us money.** Try to develop a good working relationship with your local commercial loan officer, and learn how to prepare a professional business loan application. Seek the advice of your accountant and local bookstore. Figure out alternative methods of financing. Bank of America is currently the best option for seeking this kind of financing.

Most dentists have the desire to become practice owners. For whatever the reason, a majority of dentists strive toward owning their own dental practice. Some believe that it is the only way to earn a comfortable living, while others simply do not want to be employees. It is becoming more and more difficult to own a dental practice. Many buyers of dental practices do not realize what it takes to become owner. Some don't even realize that they need to meet those monthly payments that are enabling them to put on the hat of proprietor. Sole practice owners have to worry about a lot more problems than associates do. Running a dental practice requires a lot of effort and time. The need to treat patients, and manage the business, is not an easy task. It is much more than a full time job. If you want to work less than 50 hrs per week, good luck!

If you desire to become an owner you have to realize the effort that you must put forth and you also have to learn about being a capable businessperson. Hopefully, this book will give you some of this knowledge.

Many years ago graduates could lease office space, buy equipment, put their name on a small sign, and get busy seeing patients. Those days are over! If you want to own your own dental office today, you must open up your eyes and evaluate your abilities. Patient pools are shrinking, competititon is fierce, and discretionary income is getting smaller and smaller. Managed care programs are increasing at alarming rates and taking big chunks out of our profit margins. **For now!**

If I am going to offer you one piece of advice worth the entire contents of this book it is as follows: don't wear your neighbor's old clothes! I am now in the process of building my fourth dental practice from scratch. I also owned and managed 2 medical practices and 4 other non-medical businesses. Nothin is more gratifying in life than building a multi-million dollar business from scratch. I have a negative attitude about buying an existing practice. I like to take advantage of our free enterprise system. Although "scratch" dental practices are not for everyone, you have to consider the long term profitability of owning a business that you build from nothing. Open up your own practice from scratch. Forget about buying existing practices. If you are determined enough to be your own boss you probably have an extroverted personality that will help you market to new patients and allow you to build a business in no time at all. If you have a spouse that is willing and able to help you to grow your business you will be years ahead of your competition. Follow these suggestions:

1. Choose a practical location...where you think patients need you the most, or where you can get more bang for your real estate dollar. Educate yourself on all aspects of real estate transactions (visit your local bookstore). Don't be afraid to locate in low income areas, especially if you are just starting out (you can always upgrade later). I am baffled by the number of graduates who expect to treat only fee-for-service patients in middle or upper class neighborhoods. The ignorance and short-sightedness baffles me! Practice where you are needed, or even where other professionals are afraid to go. Another helpful idea is to do some market research and look for geographic distribution of dentists in your area. Also, consult with local labs and supply houses and ask them where they feel your services may be required. If you are willing to put in long hours, accept a variety of insurance programs, and set realistic goals, you have nothing to worry about.

2. Find adequate office space and try to work out a 3 or 6 month rent deferral, unless you can purchase the property. Commercial brokers do not have multi-listings so you may have to do your own leg work and find a building that needs you. **Rent or purchase your office only where you can have at least an 8 by 10 foot internally lit sign** that says 'Dentist 555-1234' and there are a minimum of 20,000 cars going by your office daily. My first six operatory

office was 1600 square feet and it was located in a low to lower middle class neighborhood. The building was about 50 years old, but it was situated on a road that traveled over 35,000 cars per day. My sign was 8 by 10 and it was the brightest advertising in the area. I bought the building for practically nothing, renovated it, and within six months I was earning a sizable income (yes, way above the averages that are published by journal statistics). All of my friends and family thought I was crazy to open an office from scratch, especially in an area where people rode buses and lived on welfare. Five years later, I relocated to a middle class neighborhood and I am still laughing all the way to the bank. In the process I was able to pay off all of my debt, gained an immense amount of clinical experience, developed a great reputation, and build my present state-of the-art office.

3. STOP! Rethink, and begin your business plan:

* Again, look online for more information about this topic or call my office. Study all aspects of opening a business, and do not proceed until you have gained enough knowledge in this area. The Small Business Administration is also very helpful. You must do your homework. <u>Some of the most important topics are:</u>

a. Incorporation, structure of the business, tax considerations.
b. Name (choose something simple and easy to remember; if your name is Smith, call it Smith Dental and use a professional logo that your marketing company can develop.)
c. Real estate transaction (buy, rent, janitorial, repairs, maintenance, security, parking, lighting, signage, etc.). Remember, if you are not handy at doing small repairs around your home or office, rethink being an owner. Things always break and nowadays handymen are too expensive to call.
d. Preliminary financial planning and operating budget.
e. Acquire accountant, attorney, insurance agent, supplier, waste disposal, etc.
f. Telephone (start with 3 lines, 3 phones).
g. Logo, internal marketing, external marketing.
h. Staff (hire, train, motivate, etc.).
i. Bank, laboratory, referring specialists, etc.

Once you have learned about the basics of opening a new business, learn everything related to the successful management of a dental practice. Gain thorough knowledge before you spend money! Visit our website as you will find everything that you need for managing your office.

Practice management mistakes cost money, time, and effort. It is the person who prepares themselves for efficient management who will reap the rewards.

<u>Once you have finalized all legal aspects of your business, Concentrate on the following management topics:</u>

a. Communication (this book).
b. Telephone, telephone, telephone.
c. Staff training, motivation, development.
d. Cost-effective internal marketing.

e. Effective external marketing.
f. System of operations.
g. Recall system.
h. Insurance processing and collections.
i. Treatment planning.
j. Production
k. Statistics

For more info: *www.dentalofficemanagementprogram.com*

The management system available on our website is the least expensive and most comprehensive management material available on the markert. This do-it-yourself office management program will be a major asset. It's less than the cost of one crown and certainly a lot cheaper than a 7 day $30k consultant!

Another few helpful suggestions:

1. Lease 2 or 3 operatories, or purchase used equipment. Call the lease companies, or banks, in your area and see if they have any re-possesed equipment. Do not be stingy with your equipment. Fast, efficient, quality dental work requires above average dental equipment...the cost of this equipment will be negligent once you start producing profitable dentistry.
2. Answer the telephone at all hours (call forward to your house at night).
3. Return all calls by checking the caller ID (people hang up on answering machines)
4. Do your own cleanings, X-Rays, etc. until you can develop an efficient, profitable staff.
5. Carry your business card with you at all times and distribute them everywhere you go. Design a trifold, brochure style card, not a generic type.
6. Get up in the morning and distribute effective postcards or fliers to the neighborhood houses (bike-it or jog-it).
7. Purchase personalized water bottles, mugs, T-shirts and any other free gifts that you can give new patients as internal marketing pieces. Give these gifts to all of your patients after their visits; make sure you put your office name and number on the gifts!!!
8. Keep your computer system simple. Open Dental is by far the easiest and lowest cost software on the market. It's not about the bells and whistles, it's about being able to train a high school graduate on how to use your software to make appointments and bill insurance. The easier it is to learn with fewer buttons, the easier it will be to train new employees.
9. Maintain a part-time position with another office while you are getting your new place up and running.

WHAT ARE YOU EXCITED ABOUT?

WHAT ARE YOU GRATEFUL FOR?

WHAT ARE YOU PROUD OF?

WHO LOVES YOU?

WHAT DO YOU TRULY ENJOY?

HOW DO YOU FEEL?

HOW DO YOU WANT TO FEEL?

CHAPTER 9
FINANCES/MONEY

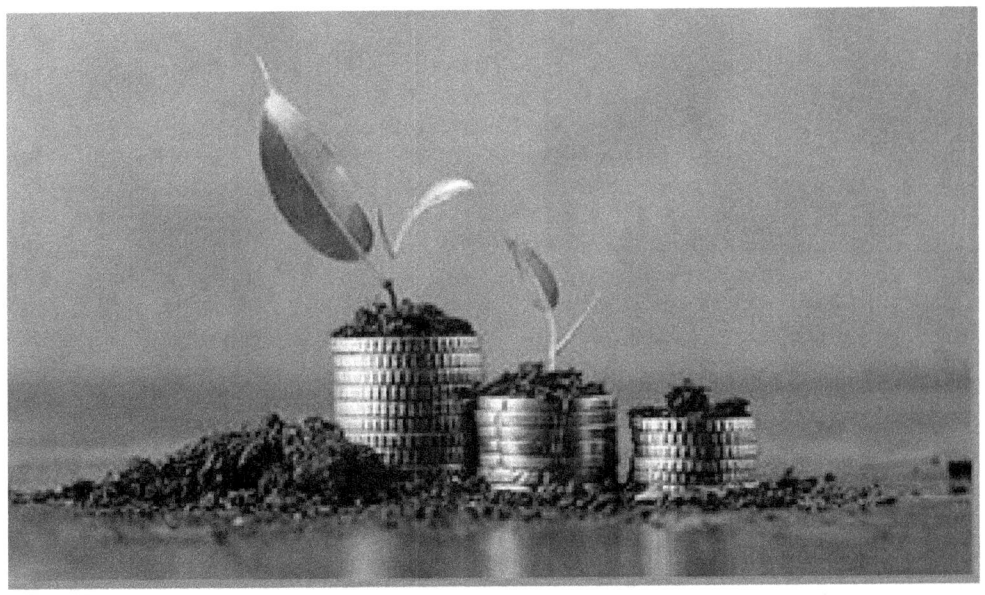

For most practitioners, accomplishment is indicated by a comfortable income. Eight years of education must be validated. The cost of your entire education was approximately $400,000. This figure, however, is grossly undervalued. Had you been working during the time that you went to school you could have easily earned approximately $400,000 (modestly earning $50,000 a year, times eight years). So you are at least $800,000 behind in income, when you compare yourself to an average paid middle class worker. **If you consider what a plumber makes, you are actually about $1,200,000 behind** (these dudes easily clear $100,000 a year). And if you decide to borrow another $500,000 to open your own office, you are now about $1,300,000 behind. Take into consideration the loss of interest earning potential for this money over a five year period, and you are now about $1,500,000 in the hole. But you have a D.D.S. or D.M.D behind your name. Yipee!

Another eye-opening fact is that your plumber and electrician friend are higher priorities in people's lives than you, the dentist. People pay the electrician and plumber before they get to your bill.

Although money should not be your main goal in life, it is somewhat important to gauge your success by financial indicators. One of the most important topics that dentists face is how much money they are going to make this year, next year, and so on!? Whether you are fresh out of school, or have been an associate or owner for many years, it is critical for you to gain knowledge of office management and finances. In order to help you realize your earning potential you must understand how a dental office operates as a business. You must understand how a dental office is managed, and you must learn your individual responsibilities that are required to make the practice efficient and profitable. Irrespective of your employment status in your practice, your income will be directly affected by your ability to understand the business protocol of the office.

Consider the demographics of our profession. There are approximately 200,000 dentists in the U.S.; roughly 70,000 dental practices. Consider another fact: Less than 10% of the U.S. population controls over 95% of the wealth. If you equate this to dentistry you can be safe to assume that 20,000 dentists, or approximately 7,000 dental practices, are controlling 95% of the "dental wealth." Are you currently one of these practitioners? Are you striving to be?

The commitment to becoming successful and wealthy requires your dedication to work toward your goals with a complete understanding of business principles and strategies. Although this chapter will not give you a masters degree in business, it will help you to realize what it takes to build a successful dental practice/career. Of course, the result of this knowledge, when applied appropriately, will directly affect your bottom line.

Like any other business, a dental office has **fixed** and **variable** expenses. The former includes costs such as rent, loan payments, telephone, contracted advertising, and other expenses that do not vary considerably from month to month. These are costs that you have to pay just to keep your front door open. The latter includes costs such as lab fees, supplies, and other expenses that can vary from month to month, depending on the number of patients treated and the number of procedures performed. Other items such as payroll, maintenance, utilities, and miscellaneous can be called borderline expenses, since they can fluctuate monthly, yet you know that they are going to be fixed, to a certain extent, due to the need to keep your front door open.

In order to understand the mechanics of operating your dental practice we will begin by discussing the need to figure out your practice's overhead.

Your starting point is to use the following formulas to...

FIGURE OUT BASIC HOURLY OVERHEAD FOR YOUR PRACTICE:

Yearly Gross ($) *divided by* 2000 hrs (normal hrs dentists work per year) = overhead per hour

or

Month Gross ($) *divided by* 166 hrs (normal hrs dentists work per month) = overhead per hour

As a general rule you must produce at least **four** times what you want to take home, if you are an associate. If you are the sole owner you have to concentrate on producing at least three times what you would like to net. If you are an owner and you have associates working for you, the scenario changes considerably, because you are using the same fixed overhead to increase production and lower total overhead. Large practices that employ multiple doctors enjoy the ability to use the same facility and the same fixed expenses to increase the amount of money that is brought in, if they are managed properly and the associates understand their individual requirement to produce dentistry at four times their take-home pay. Some large practices enjoy great profit margins as long as the employees work together to be efficient and productive. Most young dentists and recent graduates will have the experience to work for such a practice. As long as you understand your individual responsibility you can earn a comfortable income without having too many headaches.

If the hourly overhead is $200, then you must produce and collect this amount, hourly, just to pay the bills and keep the place open. Whatever you produce above this overhead figure you can start to consider as your net income. Notice that the words production and collection are inseparable. Too many management experts blow their horns telling us how much they produced. Who cares what you produce if you do not collect the same amount? Let's say that you produce/collect $2400 per day. As an associate, depending on your employment agreement with the owner, you will probably take home $800. Remember, $2400 - $800 (overhead for eight hours) = net income of $1600. Normally, $800 goes to the owner and $800 to the associate. As an owner you have taken home $1600. Of course, you have also dealt with the headaches and difficulties of running that business. As an associate you have probably left the office with a golf bag in your trunk.

Total Production - Overhead (divided by) 2 = Net Pay of an Associate (usually).
Total Production - Overhead = Net Pay of Sole Owner

Different offices use different formulas for compensation of associates. The simplest way to get paid is to receive a straight percentage of what you collect on your production. Realistically you are not going to collect 100% of what you produce. Most associates earn **30% of their collections**. This is the best way to keep it simple. Multiply your collections by **.30** and that is your take home pay. The owner may ask you to pay the same 30% of your lab fees.

Dentistry is a business. You have to start thinking like a business-person, as well as a doctor. Here are some more figures to take into account:

According to the ADA the average dentist:

Produces $550,000 per year
Works 40 hrs. per week; 49 weeks per year; 245 days per year
Has an approximate $200 per hour overhead

At the end of this chapter we will discuss some topics that will show you how to increase your profit. One of the main goals to focus on is to "think profit" during treatment planning and operative. Here's why:

A $1000 crown has a lab fee of $100 with $200 per hour overhead. If you spend one hour performing this procedure you have profitted $700. If you spend two hours, your profit is $500. Do two crowns in one hour and your profit is $1400.

A $125 composite perfomed in 45 minutes is a procedure that loses you money. 45 minutes has a $150 overhead (.75 x $200). You have lost $25. You must make it up somewhere else.

Procedure Cost - Lab Cost – (Time Spent x Overhead) = Profit

15 minutes = .25
30 minutes = .50
45 minutes = .75
60 minutes = 1.0

Learn to treatment plan full quadrant restorative, not single tooth procedures! Besides dentures, partials, crowns, bridges, and root canals there are other procedures that become very profitable, when perfomed appropriately. Extractions and composites are profitable procedures when perfomed in <u>multiple units</u>. Next time you elect not to restore the 20 year old amalgam next to the three other cavities that need restoration, think again. If you decide to place a single occlusal restoration do it at the same time that you perform your exam, radiographs, and cleaning. Don't schedule appointments for procedures that you will lose money performing. Think about your hourly overhead and your chair time! Be productive! Your bottom line profit depends on your ability to produce efficient dentistry. This, of course, does not mean quick and speedy dental work. Efficient dentistry encompasses **quality dentistry performed to the best of your abilities and at the lowest possible overhead**.

Performing quadrant dentistry is a win-win situation for both you and your patient. Get in the habit of asking your patients *"Mr. Patient would you like to complete all of the needed work in this area in one appointment, or would you like to schedule extra appointments?"*

As long as you have considered insurance coverage and patient payment ability (i.e. you have discussed your treatment plan), performing quadrant dentistry is the only way to practice dentistry. It lowers your total overhead by making your chair time efficient. Obviously your speed and clinical efficiency will have a direct effect on production and overhead. As you gain more experience and decrease the time that it takes you to complete various procedures, your profit will increase and your overhead will decrease. Concentrate on improving your techniques, working with various dental materials, eliminating failures, and completing dental work that is not in need of remake and follow-up.

QUALITY DENTISTRY TAKES TIME!

REMAKE DENTISTRY TAKES AWAY TIME, AND MONEY!

DO NOT APPOINT SINGLE LOW-COST PROCEDURES...DO THEM AT RECALLS!!!

Another aspect of maintaining profitability within an efficient practice is the requirement to **control the cost of doing business.** Before you can crack down on expenses you should familiarize yourself with an average list of dental office percentage figures of overhead. Office overhead that is above 60% is too high. Refer back to some of the following suggestions when necessary. This discussion takes into account the fact that you are an owner, or an associate, that likes to be involved in the management aspect of the business. Your accountant, or a simple business computer system such as Quickbooks, can help you get started on the track to becoming your own management consultant.

Payroll 25%
Lab 8%
Rent 7%
Supplies 5%
Marketing 5%
Misc. 5%

a. Payroll

If your figures are too high (above 25% of your gross income), check the adequacy of the work performance of your employees. Are they properly trained? Do they know how to communicate with patients? Are they enthusiastic about making the practice grow? Are they productive throughout the day? Do they take an interest in your business? Are they motivated and energetic? Do they understand the mechanics and business principles of how your practice operates?

Once you feel that your staff is properly trained, check their output. Is your schedule full and productive? Are your employees sitting around with nothing to do? Do you have too many staff members present for the amount of work that is to be done? Are a few of your employees carrying most of the work burden, while others are not? How many broken appointments do you have and why?

Begin to look at some of these areas from an outside perspective. If you come up with no solutions, then seek some outside help. Employee management is the most important aspect of running your business. Spend as much time as possible developing and training your dental team. Purchase our personnel management program online

On the contrary, if your payroll is too low (below 20% of your gross income) you should re-evaluate the compensation of your staff. You should also consider whether you may need to add employees. This could prevent potential employee burnout. Or could it be that you may be performing "non-essential" duties that an added staff member could handle?

b. Lab Cost

If your costs are escalating (above 12% of your gross income), re-evaluate your fees for procedures that involve lab cost. Your fees should be at least five times the laboratory fee. Maintain a lab log of all incoming and outgoing lab cases. At the end of the month analyze your lab expenses by tracking the various procedures performed. Adjust your fees accordingly.

You should also examine "remakes." Are you doing a lot of your work over and over? Don't run to your lab with accusations of poor workmanship. Evaluate your impression and preparation techniques. When a crown, bridge, or partial does not fit adequately it is usually a poor technique in the clinic. Rarely is it the lab technician's responsibility. Refine your techniques, check your impression trays, and update your impression material. Spend time with your local prosthodontist and lab technician!

c. Supplies

Do you maintain a well-controlled inventory system that tracks supplies as well as cost? Are you putting supplies on shelves and forgetting about them? Do you have a working relationship with a knowledgeable dental salesperson? Does your salesperson offer free incentives and free supplies when you purchase materials? Developing a good relationship with your salesperson will pay off in the long run, especially when you need supplies promptly and when returns are necessary. Your salesperson can also update you on new techniques and material, as they become available. Also, nothing wrong with shopping online such as www.net32.com

d. Rent

Are you using too much space or paying too much rent? How can you consolidate your space requirements in order to save money? On the other hand, don't get too thrifty on this expense. Adequate practice space is required in order to run a profitable business.

e. Collections

One of the most frustrating aspects of running a successful dental practice is the ability to collect what you produce. This is not always feasible since you may participate with managed care programs, or you may offer other discounts. Nevertheless, as a rule of thumb **you must collect at least 98% of your set fees**. If you participate in managed care programs, and you offer discounts, you should consider these lower fees as " write-offs" or " secondary fees," but you should not consider the reduction against your collection percentage. You should always have fee schedules set up in your sytem if you take PPOs.

Offices that have problems with collections are usually the practices where there is a lack of communication and patient education. **Do not pick up the instruments!** Do not perform dental work! Turn the compressor off...until you have discussed fees and treatment plans with your patients. In busy practices the most overlooked and neglected aspect of management is fee discussion and treatment planning. You may not always be able to do a precise treatment plan for all of your patients, since clinical treatment can involve alternatives and unforeseen problems, but you should do everything possible to finalize an agreeable treatment plan for your patients. Once you have hurdled over the obstacle of gaining your patient's trust and case acceptance you must finalize a written treatment plan that includes cost breakdown. Even if your patient has 100% insurance coverage you must do a treatment plan.

Treatment plans dictate the number of appointments, the calendar year(s) of treatment, and the patient acceptance. Patients must understand their FULL financial responsibility, along with their dental needs. If you want to offer discounts or reduced fees than you should discuss this before you begin the work. But never, ever pick up the instruments until you are sure that the patient understands their responsibility. This must happen at each and every appointment. No surprises!!!

In my opinion, if you have failed to inform your patients of the dental finances you have failed to inform them of their dental needs, as well. An informed customer is your best customer. Remember: **$200 is a lot of mullah to over 85% of the population.** Do not expect a patient to pay you $1000 for a crown if you did not quote them the fee before you began. This should also be accounted for during clinical work that includes complications (i.e. a three surface composite turning into a crown/root canal).

Always stop and review financial obligation for your patients, before you pick up the instruments and while you have picked up the instruments.

This is also very important for patients that have insurance, especially if their coverage limits or excludes any part of your proposed treatment plan. Try to collect money from someone that thought their insurance covers everything. It's what I call a lost patient! Inform before you perform! Establish the universal policy of P.A.T.O.S.: Payment At Time Of Services! **Avoid payment plans.** Get your entire staff involved in the essentials of collecting money and educating patients. Offer Care Credit and Lending Point. More about collections in the next chapter.

f. Marketing

Are you spending a lot of money on advertising, while forgetting the back door phenomenon? Always track the amount of money that you spend to bring patients to your office. Include a sentence on your health history for the patient to advise you about how they heard of your practice. Track these expenses monthly and figure out your return on investment. Spend money strictly on the marketing avenues that bring in the most amount of patients for the least amount of money.

A large sign should be your number one advertising. If your practice is on a well traveled road, a simple sign that reads: "Dentist 555-1234" is all that is necessary to bring in new patients.

If you want to expand your marketing to include direct mail, seek the help of a professional who will help you design an effective marketing piece. Do not rush and spend thousands of dollars on an amateur flier or postcard. Let the pros handle it for you. Your investment will result in a much higher reward. Call us for more advice. This is a topic covered in large volumes.

Keep these basics in mind when marketing your practice:

* A professional website and Google Business Listing are your Number 1 forms of advertising. Don't spend money anywhere else until you hire the right company to manage this aspect.

* Facebook and Instagram can be very powerful if done from a personal perspective. Same company can do this for you.

* Nothing wrong with Snail Mail Advertising. Full-color 6 x 4 postcards are very noticeable. Use professional photos to liven up the advertising piece. Visite www.postcardmania.com They have beautiful marketing postcards.

* Always include a financial advantage for the reader to visit your practice (i.e. *exam, Bitewings, and cleaning for $95 and Guaranteed, Complete Bleaching for $95)*. Give away the visit if you have to. Your goal is to get patients through your door and develop a long term relationship with them, as well as their extended family and friends. Your internal marketing will take over and these new patients will act as missionaries for your office. Once they have a great experience at your office they will tell all of their friends and family. Obviously you will also discover many dental problems and cosmetic needs that will make your low-fee visit profitable once you get to do all of that nice dentistry.

* List the ways you deal with fearful patients and busy schedules *(i.e. we provide gentle, non-hurried, modern care that meets your schedule and your budget)*. Remember: all people want to avoid pain and gain pleasure!

* Don't forget to list all possible credentials that you and any of your staff members have (list all licenses and memberships you have, as well as organizations that you belong to). A photo of you and/or your staff is a good idea, as long as it is professionally produced.

* Other professionally produced photos are also encouraged. Family type poses are highly effective. Videos are even better.

* Do not list dental procedures, such as root canals or fillings or gum treatments. These elicit sensations of pain in people's minds. Patients respond positively to emotions of pleasure, not pain. That's why you should let the pros handle your ads.

* End all of your advertising with a call to action, "CALL TODAY 555-1234."

Whenever I ask a colleague how they market their practices I usually hear the same type of answer: "Well, I have a website and I send out fliers." It is rare that I hear anybody tell me how they market themselves, their staff, and their practice.

To be successful in dentistry you must learn to market yourself, first and foremost. Reading this book is the starting point to making yourself marketable. Your people skills, clinical skills, and atitude will help you promote - YOU. Patients that like you as a person, and as a dentist, will tell their friends and family members. This is the best advertising that you can develop. A few other things you should get in the habit of doing are very simple and basic.

First, carry your business card at all times. Give it to everyone you meet. Make sure your card is designed to list more than just your name and number. Put a coupon, or other benefit, that motivates the recipient to call your office. My business card has my photo, my credentials, benefits of coming to our office, and a coupon for free exam and X-rays. It is designed, like a brochure, to help motivate the holder into picking up the phone and making an appointment.

Second, learn to ask patients to refer their family and friends. Do so especially with the patients that you like. Flocks of a feather stick together! Don't sound desperate. Use the following phrase: ***"Mr. Jones, we really enjoy having you as a patient at our office and we would like to see more of your friends and family."*** It is always helpful to personally ask your valued patients for more referrals. Patients usually forget about you once they leave the office (unless they're in pain...ha - ha) but if you make it a point to ask them to refer their family and friends, then you may actually get them talking to people about you and about their good experiences at your office. Asking for referrals should never take on a desperation tone: "We need more patients, we hope you can refer some people to our office!" This is a sure way to lose trust from your patients.

Teach your front desk the following dialogue:

"Mrs. Smith, I take it your visit today was pleasant and comfortable as always. (if yes..) I'm real happy to hear that and I hope that if any of your friends or family require our services you would pass along our business card to them, or better yet I can always arrange a free visit for them as long as you would like us to...just have them remind me that they are your friend or family and I will make sure that there is no charge for their exam."

If you want, you can also give the patient the same coupon that may have brought them into the office.

On the other side of the ocean, Never be ungrateful when patients ask you to see their friend or relative. The phrase *"We're very busy but I guess we can squeeze your mother in"* should never come out of your mouth. Instead...*"Oh, of course, Mrs. Smith we would be delighted to see your mother at our office. Just let me know what is a convenient time to schedule an appointment for her and I will make sure that her first office visit is free of charge!"*

Another great approach to stimulating even more referrals is to make the patient active in the referral process. Patients of record, especially those who maintain good dental health, are a great source of education for other people in the community. Talk to these patients about their ability to make a positive impact for somebody else:

"Mrs. Smith, you have taken good care of your dental health for a long time and I'm sure you know just as we do that there are a lot of people out there that simply do not take the time to care for their teeth, or their health, the way you do. We normally like to ask patients such as yourself to educate other people on the benefits of modern dentistry and medicine. A lot of people don't visit our office until they are in pain...and this visit usually involves somewhat uncomfortable, expensive treatment. If you know someone like that please refer them to us and explain to them the benefits of preventive medicine and dentistry."

One of the best ways I have found to keep patients talking about me and my practice is to provide ALL patients with gifts such as mugs, T-shirts, dinners, water bottles, etc. At my office ALL patients receive free water bottles, coffee mugs, travel mugs, balloons, brushes, sugarless candy, and other promotional gizmos that we can stuff in a customized, plastic bag. Of course, my practice name and phone number are on all of them, including the bag.

Frequent referrers receive a steak dinner, or tickets to the movies.

We also like to offer $60 same as cash towards future dental work for each and every referral. We have some patients that have accumulated thousands of dollars in credits due to their referrals. Consults do NOT count towards this credit. Remember, that you are most likely spending over $100 in advertising cost for each New Patient. $60 is a lot cheaper and you will get better patients.

It's amazing how other kids want to become patients at our office when they see our kids playing with the toys and baloons that they just received after their cleaning. This is true when children leave the office and stop by at McDonald's, or other fast food restaurants. What a great way to market the practice, for a few pennies!

Once you have marketed yourself, you have also marketed your office. Your staff should also help to market you and your practice. All members should have their own business cards and/or yours. They should distribute brochures and literature to all patients, as well as their friends and family. The more literature that leaves your office, the more that you and your practice will benefit.

Other marketing ideas can be implemented if you are trying to build clientele. The simpler you keep these advertising avenues the more response you will receive. Here's a few other helpful ideas:

1. Work evening hours and Saturdays.
2. Call-forward your telephone to your house after hours (put in a second line).
3. Get caller I.D. for your telephone.
4. Market to new residents
5. Send birthday cards to your patients.

6. Send newsletters to all of your patients (include referral cards, bleaching coupons, or any other promotions that you may want to advertise).
7. Avoid TV, Radio, and Newspaper advertising.
8. Call the local media if you are implementing a new technique, or product, in your practice. Get free news publicity.
9. Use profesionally produced videos to educate your patients.
10. Follow-up with a Thank-You-For-Choosing-Our-Office Postcard to all new patients. Handwrite it!
11. Get involved in the lives of your patients. If someone is sick, send them a get-well gift basket of your liking. If someone accomplishes a milestone in their lives, send them a card or gift (i.e. 50th wedding anniversary, college graduation, high school graduation, work promotion, etc.). Keep an open eye and interest in the lives of your patients.

To conclude this chapter, I would like to open up your eyes a little and make you realize that there is money in dentistry. You will hear many of your colleagues scorn, complain, and bicker about being a dentist. This is normal. Dentistry is a hard profession, emotionally as well as physically and mentally. At the same time, dentistry can provide you with a good living, great working hours, and a lot of flexibility.

After I graduated from dental school I bought and read every financial and business book I could get my hands on. I knew that I wanted to own my own practice. I also realized that I needed to sharpen my business skills, financial knowledge, and human relations abilities before opening up my own place.

You have to consider being financially stable within ten years of graduation from dental school. After seven years of being out of dental school I could have easily sold all of my dental assets and retired with a nice nest egg.

As a new associate who is fresh out of school you should be earning about $100,000 a year during your first two years. After two years you should be earning about $150,000 a year. As an owner, you should be taking home at least $250,000, if you have more than 1,000 active patients. Obviously the part of the country where you live will affect these numbers!

Couple this earning potential with the ability to use your business write-offs and you should realize that dentistry is a profitable business.

DON'T EXPECT MONEY TO BUY YOU HAPPINESS

REAL SUCCESS IS PEACE, HEALTH, AND LOVE

CHAPTER 10
STAFF RELATIONS

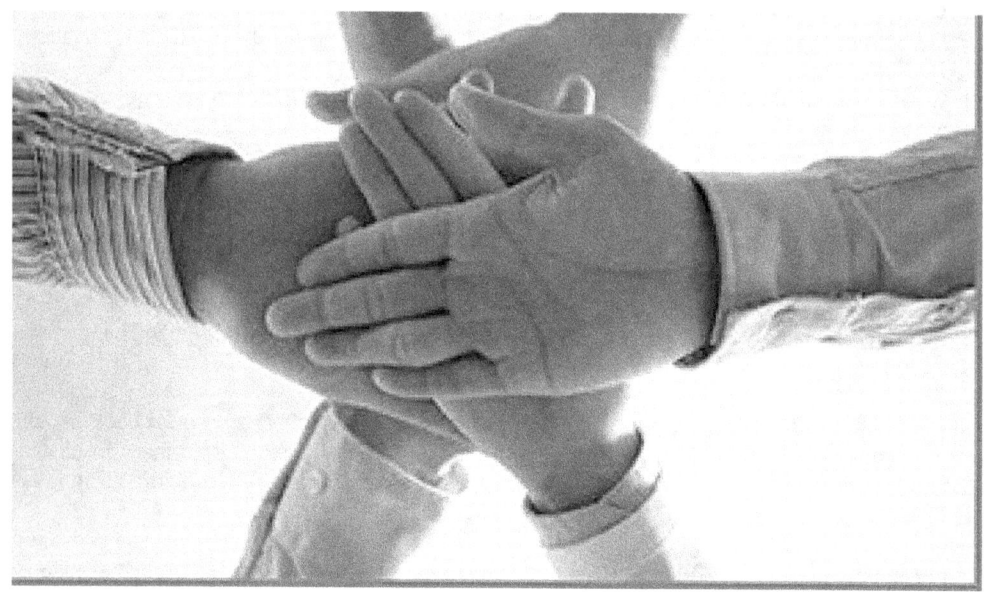

Your progress in dentistry will either be facilitated or hampered by the people that surround you. Owners and associates must discipline themselves in terms of gaining knowledge and expertise in the area of employee management. Learn to improve your people relations skills and the persons around you will help you to reach your goals. The staff that you will work with will be the determining factor for your success. You have to educate yourself on the legalities of employment and you have to improve your staff relations skills. Here is an excerpt from one of the articles that I have written in the past:

MOTIVATING AND MANAGING YOUR EMPLOYEES

An evaluation of the motivation and performance of today's work force would reveal that businesses all over the country are plagued with careless attitudes and sub-standard work output. Is your practice becoming one of these statistics? Inadequate employee work performance is limiting your personal and practice growth. To combat this problem you must take control of your business and begin managing your employees.

You must do everything possible to help your employees achieve their full potential. Your team members are your most important asset and payroll is the largest portion of your overhead. A well-trained and supervised staff will make an average practice successful. It is your responsibility to hire, train, and manage your team to maximize daily output.

Poor employee work performance is a result of a lack of motivation. This problem can be solved by improving staff morale and inspiration. Easily said, hard to accomplish! Motivation, enthusiasm, and optimistic attitudes cannot be created as easily as some may believe. Most psychology experts agree that motivation is located internally...you either have it or you don't. Despite this fact, you can still follow certain protocols to nurture motivation and prevent wearisome employee attitudes.

Just how do you get your employees to do what you want them to do? "How do I motivate my employees to get things done?" Rule #1: realize the work benefits that are most important to your employees (refer to the seven basics listed below). Rule #2: implement a system of communication and employee work performance feedback, as described below. Once you begin to follow some of the following suggestions, your employee motivation will improve due to the fact that you are implementing a system of human relations that is geared towards the needs of your staff.

Today's employee is looking for more than just a boss who can provide them with a good salary.

Your employees want:

1. To be appreciated.
2. To have flexible hours.
3. To be involved and be able to make decisions.
4. To have job security.
5. To have good wages.
6. To have interesting work.
7. To have good working conditions and good equipment.

Refer to these seven benefits as often as possible!!!

Employees want to have a challenging job that provides them with the independence to decide how to do their work. Once this work is completed they expect to be noticed and appreciated. When is the last time you told one of your staff members "Thank you, nice job!"? Bonuses and monetary compensation are not as important to quality employees as is appreciation and autonomy. Allow your staff to decide how to do their work and appreciate their efforts and performance.

Employees search for jobs that provide flexibility. Allow your staff to be able to take care of their personal needs. Let your employees help you decide their working hours and even have input on your office schedule. Provide your employees with flexible hours. They will have other needs to meet besides their job duties. Flexibility on your behalf means a lot to your workers. You should also consider allowing employees to finish some of their work at home (i.e. billing, collections, recalls).

Your team members want to make sure that their next paycheck is not going to do a crazy-ball bounce. Is your business struggling? Does everybody feel secure and comfortable? Employees will search for other jobs if you show signs of business troubles. They want security and peace of mind. Get your business in tip-top shape and never share financial concerns or business woes with your employees. Don't rock the boat!

Are you paying your employees with peanuts and expecting them to lay golden eggs? Check your employee wages against similar jobs in other fields and in the dental industry. Match and exceed those averages as much as possible.

Are your employees satisfied with their jobs? Could it be possible that their work is getting boring and monotonous? Do they communicate their concerns to you? Do you have an open door policy to receive staff input? Communication between you and your staff is an essential component of developing your staff relations. Conduct frequent staff analysis, in writing. Develop forms that allow your employees to share their thoughts with you. Use some of the following sentences in your forms:

1. What do you enjoy most about your job?
2. What do you dislike about your job?
3. What suggestions do you have for improving the working conditions in the office?
4. What suggestions do you have for improving our relationship with patients?
5. Do you find your work interesting and challenging?
6. How do you feel about your co-workers?
7. How do you like to be appreciated?
8. What would you like your boss to change?

Your employees will let you know how they feel. Welcome all comments. Don't let your feelings be hurt. Your team members will give you honest feedback and provide great business insight for your office. They will tell you how to improve your staff relations and your practice protocols better than anyone else. All you have to do is listen and take criticism and suggestions constructively. Make sure to act upon these suggestions and make changes accordingly.

Provide your employees with all of the necessary equipment, surroundings and supplies that they need to perform their duties. These items include such basics as good lighting, modern equipment, comfortable temperature, ergonomically designed chairs, a lunch area, clean bathrooms, and other tangibles that your employees may request. Acknowledge the efforts and accomplishments of your staff and supply them with a great working environment.

Besides the above employee relations criteria, you must take the time to provide your team members with continuous objective feedback and evaluation. This should be done in writing on a quarterly basis. Your employees should be allowed to complete their own evaluation before you do your analysis. The employee evaluation is a tool for improving communication and solving problems. Feedback is the only tool that you have to assess the function of your operations. It is also critical in developing the work performance and future output of your employees. Design your own evaluation forms, if necessary. Keep them objective and specific. Try to cover specific analysis for all job duties.

At least one hour should be set aside for every employee when it comes time to discuss your review. As you complete the employee analysis do not dwell on negatives. Stress positive work performance and avoid accusatory language. Phrases such as "I feel that...," or "I don't believe that...," should never be included in your discussions. Never be vague! Do not fear discussion of poor work output. Deficiencies should be addressed as shortcomings that need improvement, training, or further education. At the conclusion of the evaluation schedule training or continuing education seminars for areas of work performance that are lacking. Have employee sign the evaluation and place it in his/her personnel file.

Allow the following sentence to be integrated into your evaluations and into your everyday analysis of employee work performance: "Your work performance is extremely good when you..." Obviously you must continuously fill-in-the blank with the duties that you want your employees to perform to the best of their abilities.

Allow yourself to be evaluated!!! Take comments with a positive attitude. Make appropriate changes. Do not procrastinate. A pleasant working environment starts with the doctor. The staff is usually an extension of the doctor. Do not be afraid to be the focal point. Maintain an open door policy to suggestions and input from your staff. Carry yourself by exhibiting happiness and optimism. Smile, laugh, and be productive.

Your team members will use the owner (and/or manager) as a focal point for their professional development. Are you providing a good work example to your employees? Are you fair in your decisions? Are you objective in your employee analysis? Do you provide training? Do you emphasize continuing education? Do you take an interest in the personal life and well-being of your employees? Do you handle problems and conflicts with calm and tact? Do you let your staff know how important they are to you? Do you give credit and recognition often?

Reward your staff with security, good wages, and an open attitude towards future change. Your staff is your biggest asset. Treat your employees according to how you want your office to function. Once the above criteria have been met, implement a bonus system based on efficiency and productivity. This bonus system should take into account employee work performance, collections, practice building, and expense control. It should not consider increases in production, patient numbers, or collections without observing overhead control and cost overruns.

In conclusion, follow these basic factors for improving your staff motivation and development:

1. Allow employees to be independent and solve problems on their own.
2. Allow employees to complete tasks without your help.
3. Provide interesting work and try to change the way you do things.
4. Receive and provide continuous input from/for your employees.
5. Provide your employees with safe surroundings and adequate equipment.

Your staff is your biggest asset. You must ask yourself daily **"What have I done and what can I do to improve my staff?"** The staff you work with will willingly help you to achieve your daily objectives if you remember to refer to some of the above ideas and suggestions.

If you are hired as an associate you will have to overcome the obstacle of molding with the current staff. Many times this involves adaptation on both sides of the court. Although you should stick to your guns and do things the way you would like to have them done, be open minded to suggestions and education. Most staff members do not want to change their routines and operations for you. Learn to accept this fact. Welcome input in regard to how you should do things. You may be pleasantly surprised when a veteran staff member will show you a few things that dental school never taught you.

A well-trained staff is a priceless commodity. Many dental offices suffer from high turn-over rates of employees. Although this change may never be adequately controlled, **you should do your share to help decrease the effects of staff turn-over.**

First, maintain an open eye for potential future employees at all times. Almost anyone with the right attitude and skills can be trained to work in a dental office. Encourage friends, acquaintances, and even family members to consider a career in dentistry.

Second, try to maintain part-time employees that are flexible to cover during periods of change. Finally, realize the benefits of maintaining a stable, well-trained staff.

If you own your own practice please consider investing in our management system. There is a lot more information that you need to learn, on this topic, in order to manage your staff and achieve optimal performance.

A system of operations is critical to the survival and profitability of any business, especially a dental office. Once you have an efficient MS (Management System) you will see employee morale improve, staff turnover decrease, and profit margins increase. Without a good MS your business will always struggle. Our MS costs less then a crown fee and will give your business more information than any expensive consultant can ever provide for you and your practice.

Our DO IT YOURSELF OFFICE MANAGEMENT PROGRAM is a must for any practitioner who owns a practice or wants to see their practice succeed.

SUCCESS CAN ONLY BE ACHIEVED WHEN ALL PARTS WORK TOGETHER

CHAPTER 11
COMMON-SENSE EXPERTISE

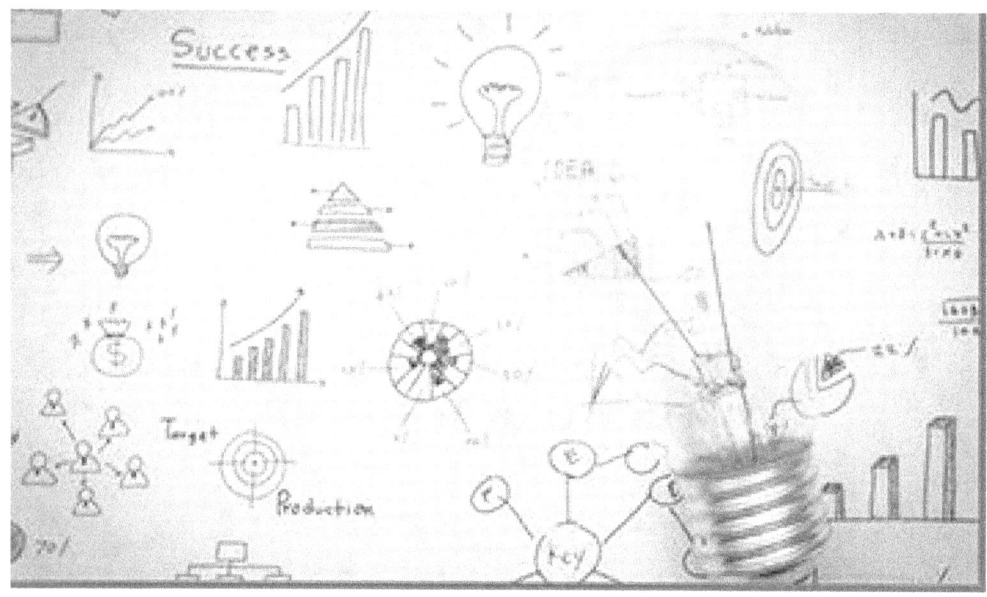

Clinical skills take time to develop! People skills take time to develop! Before you can build a successful career, and become a top-notch practitioner, **you must be a great communicator and an excellent clinician**. Dentistry is a complex science that involves an immense amount of expertise, knowledge, and ability. First, you must be able to present it to your patients and then you must be able to provide it to your patients. There is no value in the ability to provide quality dental care if you cannot educate your patients and help them to perceive the value of their dental needs. The practitioner who wants to perform quality dental care must master the art of communication and human relations.

Daily, in my practice, I see a lot of dentistry that belongs in the waste receptacle. I have come to know some of my patient's previous dentist by simply looking at the dental work performed in their mouth. Although many of us have a "bad" day now and then, there are some practitioners who have continuously lousy days. I have known many practitioners that can barely complete a Class I amalgam, yet have incredible communication abilities and are able to motivate their patients into accepting necessary treatment. Of course there are those practitioners who possess great communication abilities and awesome clinical skills.

Even the best of us will not always perform acceptable dentistry...we would not be human if we were constantly perfect. Do not hold yourself to standards of perfection - you will go bonkers!!! However, do everything possible to become a good clinician and provide your patients with a service that is worthy of the hard earned money that they are paying you. Learn to diagnose, treatment plan, educate, and perform.

Have pride in your work, and substantiate the cost of your services. If you have a bad day, now and then, don't be afraid to become your worst critic. Communicate and be truthful to your patients! Don't hide mistakes or poor workmanship...it could come back to haunt you! Always remake below average procedures. Get used to the following phrase because you will need to use it once in a while: *"Mr. Patient, the _____ that I just completed on this tooth does not meet my expectations for quality dental work. I will need to remake it so that it will last you many years!"* If you cannot remake the work, refer! But never hide anything!

Your <u>average</u> patient cannot afford dental care in excess of $2000. One crown is an astronomical expense to most of your patients. It is up to you to inform your patient of their need, build value for the need, motivate them to accept treatment, and complete their dentistry with above average results.

Before you can learn to expand your clinical abilities, you must realize one very important concept: nobody cares how much you know, but they know how much you care. In order to get to do dental work for your patients you must develop excellent communication skills, appropriate bed-side manners, and empathy. These go hand in hand with another concept: your professional success depends on how much people like and trust you. You don't have to look like a movie star to get people to like you and feel comfortable with you. You must, however develop a few people skills that will help you to achieve case acceptance and patient trust.

The rest of this book will cover information to help build upon your dental school education. They are based upon my clinical experience, patient contact, and knowledge of the dental profession. Adapt these suggestions to your development as best as you can. Good communication and clinical skills lead to profit and less stress! Poor communication and clinical skills lead to high overhead, negative marketing, legal problems, and personal set-backs.

SUCCESS DOES NOT FIND YOU - YOU MUST FIND IT

CHAPTER 12
STOP - A WORD ABOUT EXPERTS

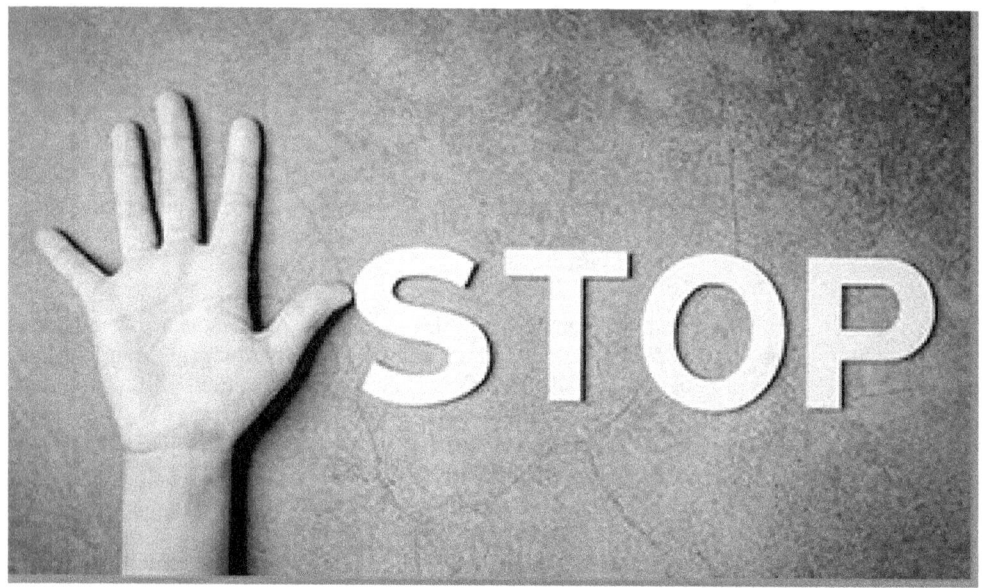

This book is written from a practical, no nonsense viewpoint. It is basically my conception of what it takes to become successful in dentistry. Adapt any of my suggestions to your own personal style. If they don't work, try again. If they still don't work, ask yourself why they are not working. Try again and if you still don't succeed, then maybe you should try a different approach. I am not an expert in human relations, communication, or clinical dentistry. What I am sharing with you is what I have found useful and practical in **my** approach with patients. What works for you may be totally different. It is helpful to remember this suggestion whenever you receive any type of advice from anyone, especially the so-called experts.

Successful people do not rely on advice from experts and specialists.

They use common sense and sensibility, mixed with ideas and suggestions from others.

They don't need experts to tell them what works and what does not. I am by no means an expert and you should never consider anyone else to be such a person.

This is especially true when you go to seminars and lectures. I see too many dentists trying to emulate the so-called gurus of dentistry. If you only knew the real truth behind some of these professionals you would probably never go to another seminar. Learn things with a grain of salt from seminar speakers and don't get too brainwashed by what they tell you. Always ask yourself, " If this person is so successful why is he/she living out of a hotel room trying to tell me how to run my career?"

In the long run, you are your own best, expert.

WHAT HAPPENS TO A PERSON IS LESS SIGNIFICANT THAN WHAT HAPPENS WITHIN THAT PERSON

HOW AND WHAT YOU FEEL ABOUT YOURSELF DICTATES YOUR WHOLE LIFE

DEFINE YOURSELF

CHAPTER 13
COMMUNICATION/HUMAN RELATIONS

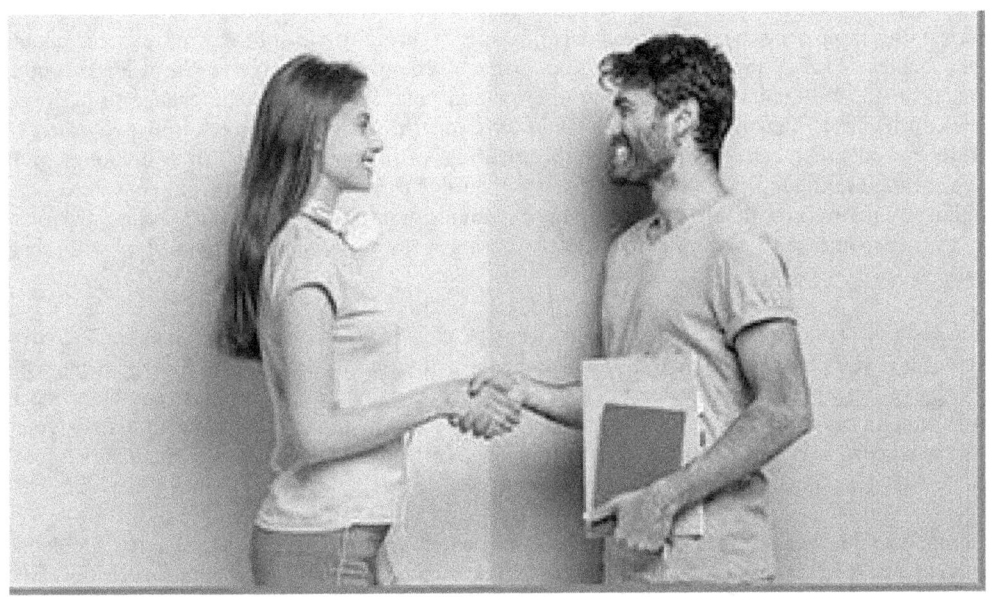

I hired an associate a few years ago who's clinical skills were, for the most part - atrocious. This "doctor" could not even finish decay removal for an occlusal amalgam. He was simply a lousy dentist. I knew I could not keep him in the office, due to the fact that I was constantly re-doing his work and bailing him out of tough situations. But I observed one important characteristic that this guy possessed. He had superb communication skills. Patients loved him, listened to him, and were motivated into treatment by his communication skills. Patients trusted him. So I let him sell dentistry and treatment plans. I had him present optimal treatment and he stressed the referral of the patient into my expertise. Soon enough, I was performing an increased amount of crown and bridge. Some of this work I had previously presented to my patients without much acceptance.

Along the way I learned one thing from my experience with a lousy dentist: <u>effective communication is the key to success</u>. I began to develop my communication skills more. Also, I quickly came to realize that my patient relations were improving, while my bottom line was becoming lean and mean. I began to see dentistry from the patient perspective and started to tailor my approach towards the personality, perception, and needs of the patient. This took place with the desire to improve my communication skills.

To succeed in any area of your professional or personal life you must learn to communicate effectively.

Communication is the cornerstone of successful people. Communication is defined by the dictionary as the exchange of thoughts, messages, etc. It is the foundation of your personal development and growth. To become a successful dentist you have to realize that you must improve your communication skills.

The ability to provide dental services depends upon your ability to inform your patients about their dental needs. Without informing your patients they will not perceive the value of good dental health. Without this exchange of information you will not have the chance to perform clinical dentistry. **You must get yourself away from thinking about teeth and procedures. Rather, you must concentrate on communicating with your patients, in a personal and professional manner.** It is the only way you will be able to build trust, gain case acceptance, and ultimately perform profitable dentistry. This communication process must start during your first patient encounter and continue indefinitely during your professional relationship with that patient.

Your purpose is to provide care for your patients. Obviously you are dealing with the oral cavity, however if you limit your expertise to this area you will fail as a professional. Your patients will bring their emotions into your trust. Teeth are a secondary purpose. You must be able to deal with unique personalities and different emotional needs. In order to be able to satisfy your patient's needs you must learn how to communicate effectively. Without communication, your professional and personal development will stagnate.

Communication helps you to develop excellent people relations skills and effective problem-solving abilities. Therefore, effective communication helps you deal with patients, staff members, and other people in your life. Your people/patient service will be greatly improved and your life will be less stressful. Developing communication skills will make you a people professional.

In school you enjoyed talking and educating patients because it was exciting, new and challenging. Most of the time you actually enjoyed hearing yourself talk about the things you were learning. **As years go by in private practice the daily pressures and constant demands will erode the quality of your communication. You will find yourself leaving out simple and important words and phrases in order to speed up your work schedule and see more patients. You will begin to shortcut your explanations thereby diminishing the effectiveness of your communication.** Your patients will not receive the entire picture because you will be assuming that they understand what you're trying to say.

I recently had a patient come to the office wanting to have her entire dentition restored. After doing all of the appropriate work-up I explained everything that she needed to have done. This included bite appliance therapy, periodontal surgery, root canals, cores, and multiple crowns and bridges. It took me about ten minutes to explain this to her. A week later she came in for her appointment to have the periodontal treatment commenced. She looked at me and said "So what are we going to do with my mouth?" I just about threw myself through the window. After I calmed down I realized that the ten minute consultation was simply not enough time to explain a complex treatment plan to this patient. I had missed too many important details and aspects of treatment. I did not communicate effectively with this patient. I did not address her needs, whether perceived or real. I failed this patient. I was surprised that she even showed up for her next appointment.

Inconsistent patient education leads to decreased case acceptance, decreased appointments, increased broken appointments, collections problems, and staff turnover. Your self esteem will suffer once you begin to doubt yourself and the trust that patients are placing in you. Stress will happen (remember Chapter 6?).

Before you can begin to develop effective people skills you must become flexible and versatile. The reason for the need to be adaptable is due to the fact that there are four basic personality types amongst all people. You must learn to understand and differentiate between these personalities in order to appreciate the variance between people. You must learn these different personalities in order to adjust your approach and communication skills. Although during a busy schedule you cannot always become a psychologist, you should have a basic knowledge of the basic personality temperaments. They are as follows:

EXPRESSIVE - a friendly, cheerful person who is animated, humorous, and spontaneous.

These patients like quick and orderly presentations. They like small talk, humor, and do not care about facts and details. They tend to be disorganized, undisciplined and restless.

DRIVER - a non-emotional person who is impatient, stubborn, and likes to take charge.

This patient likes to have options so that they can make the decision. They do not like too many details and can be obnoxious.

ANALYTICAL - a cautious person who likes to be a perfectionist that dwells on being picky, critical, and technical.

This patient loves details, pros/cons, facts, alternatives, technicalities of treatment. They can also be very sensitive.

AMIABLE - a soft-hearted person who is happy, loyal, supportive, reliable, unselfish, and happy.

This patient likes re-assurance, soft approach, and your interest in their personal life. They can also be too laid back and lazy.

Patients choose to proceed with their dental work if you have met their emotional, intellectual, and psychological needs. Three out of four of your patients will not care about what is involved in the actual process of completing their dental work. Only one out of four will be interested in the mechanics of dentistry and take the time to listen to your procedural explanations. In order to help you deal with different people, and their varying personalities, you must learn to adapt your communication skills and case presentation approach.

You have been taught to diagnose and provide ideal dentistry. In order to be able to do this, you must sell it through effective communication. Effective communication leads to proper patient education and therefore establishes value for your services. Most dental practices have about a 68% case acceptance rate. This is an extremely low number and it is due to the fact that **people do not value what they do not understand and will not buy what they do not value.**

It is up to you to create value!

As you develop your people skills you will come to realize that you can safely begin to categorize your patients, to a certain extent. Most people will give you an insight into their personality, either through physical attributes or external demeanor. Pay attention to gestures and body mannerism. Be aware of patient's conduct, attitude, behavior, dress, and overall appearance. A " driver" may be a business owner who insists upon quick appointments. He/she may be dressed in a business suit or even casual clothes. An " analytical" may be wearing your typical nerd look. An " amiable" may be dressed in any fashion and usually has a pleasing behavior. An "expressive" patient most likely wears the latest fashion and likes to attract attention.

Try to pick out some physical attribute in order to help you adapt to the patient's personality style. Of course this is not always possible, so the following suggestions will help you adapt an approach that is cross-sectioned for all of these groups.

One of the most important aspects of your patient communication process is to look for such defensive signs as folded arms, fidgety hands, cold sweating, wandering eyes, irritability, etc. These patients will need a lot of education and empathy. Once you make people feel comfortable dealing with them will become easier and your professional growth will never stagnate.

ALL of your patients will have four basic concerns when they visit your office:

1. **FEAR (an emotional and psychological factor).**
2. **MONEY**
3. **TIME AWAY FROM WORK**
4. **OUTCOME OF TREATMENT (esthetics, comfort, longevity, etc.)**

Most patients are not concerned about your materials and your procedures. They want to know how much it's going to hurt, how expensive the treatment will be, how much work they will have to miss, and how their teeth will feel and look when you're done. These are the things that people **value** in terms of their dental needs. This is all that your patients will concern themselves with. **Meet your patients' needs by addressing their concerns!** Develop communication skills geared towards addressing your patient's concerns and providing answers to their questions.

Do not suffocate patients with what you know they need to have done. Tailor your approach to meeting their personal perception of their needs. Slowly, begin your education process and establish value for optimal care. For example, a patient wants a cleaning and you have just diagnosed Moderate Periodontitis. Don't schedule an appointment for root planing without taking the time to explain to the patient why a cleaning is not possible. Take the extra ten minutes, show a video, go over brochures, and educate the patient. Once the patient realizes how they will benefit from treatment and how they will avoid future pain, cost, and loss of teeth they will see the value of the treatment and be eager to have it completed.

You cannot use the same educational approach with different people. You must learn to distinguish amongst different personalities in order to become an effective communicator and "salesperson". Here are some basics:

1. **All** patients should receive a treatment plan, financial responsibility explanation, consent form, and advantages/disadvantages of treatment. The rest of your approach in dealing with patients relies upon your case presentation. More on this subject in later chapters.

2. **Directive personalities** should receive quick recommendations that stress examples of similar dental work. Show brief examples of other patient's dental work that is similar to theirs. Be brief and to the point. Stress advantages/disadvantages of treatment. Allow patient to make up their own mind!

3. **Expressive personalities** should receive a lot of attention from you and your entire staff. Talk about the weather and the patient's interests. Stress cosmetic work and explain to this patient how spending the money for the dental work will benefit their health, looks, and comfort. Show similar dental work with lots of visual material. Give this patient brochures and any office internal marketing gifts you may have.

4. **Analytical personalities** like to discuss details and specifics. Explain dental procedures with all of the technicalities included. Take time to explain your treatment plan and listen attentively, without being in a hurry. Reassure the patient by following up in a few weeks with a telephone call, in case they do not schedule for necessary treatment. Make sure your written material is neat and organized. Remember something personal about this patient. Talk slowly!

5. The **amiable personality** is a lot like the analytical except that they do not care about the technical stuff. They need reassurance and want you to help them make up their mind. Don't be afraid to go to the front desk and personally schedule their next appointment.

One of the most important aspects of communicating with your patients is to LISTEN and not be in a rush. Most practitioners feel that they should do most of the talking while presenting a treatment plan, in order to " speed" things up. You must guard yourself against this belief and habit, if you desire to gain case acceptance and patient trust. Never be in a rush to present optimal treatment plans and allow your patients to do most of the talking. If you try to develop one skill in the next twelve months it should be to listen. Great ears and an open mind will help you become a great communicator. Here are a few suggestions to help you become a great listener. **THE L.A.D.D.E.R. TECHNIQUE:**

Listen attentively by consuming yourself with what the other person has to say
Ask questions to help you make sure that you understand everything being said
Don't interrupt
Don't judge what the other person is saying (accept other views)
Empathize
Respond with positive remarks that help elicit further communication

Listening will help you become a better dentist, better employer, better parent, better friend, and better person.

Most people will come to you with a problem. They're not only asking for advice, but also asking for your attention and care. You must listen in order to gain their trust and provide them with your dental expertise.

Get out of the following habits:

1. Offering quick solutions and advice (take the time to find out what the patient thinks they need and what they want to have done).
2. Preaching and criticizing.
3. Making fun of someone's problem.

Develop the following habits:

1. Try to develop a slow approach based on establishing good eye contact. This is best achieved by picking a spot in between the person's eyes and focusing on this area (don't try to look directly into a person's eyes as they speak; it will make both of you uncomfortable). Inadequate eye contact indicates distrust, intimidation, or insecurity. Soft approach with unobtrusive eye contact!!!

2. Shake your head in agreement to show that you are paying attention. Paraphrases, such as "I see," "Tell me more," "Go on," "I'd like to know more," will invite further discussion. Silence is golden! Learn this principle, **especially when dealing with irate or angered people.**

3. Observe the other person's gestures and body movements. Don't cross your arms! Maintain positive facial expressions. Pay attention to signs of nervousness coming from the other side. Patients that tug at their ears, raise their eyebrows, fidget, or otherwise appear squeamish are expressing a feeling of doubt or insecurity. Reassure all of these patients by allowing them to express their thoughts and feelings. Re-emphasize your previous statements and/or repeat their sentences to make sure that you heard what they were trying to say.

4. Imitate and/or mirror the person, <u>in a discreet and non-apparent manner</u>. If they want to stand up out of the chair, you should do likewise. If they inter-twine their fingers, do likewise. If they place their arms on their hips, do likewise. I think you get the point!

5. Be modest. Let others toot their horn; unplug yours.

6. Accept people for what they are, not what you think they should be.

7. Get your staff involved in the communication process and continuously update this requirement.

The last part of communication deals with word and sentence choice. You must develop these skills on your own. Attempt to keep your language simple and logical. Don't blow away your patients with words like "obturation," "debridement," "tapered preparation," etc. Keep your language simple and common.

Include the **"feel, felt, thought"** strategy in your communication process. *"Mrs. Patient, I understand how you feel about your teeth, and I can help you with the best treatment for your teeth because it will be a life-time decision and investment that you will be making."*

Remember the empathizing part of communication. Show people that you understand their feelings and that you will provide them with what's necessary because _____.

<u>Don't</u> get in the habit of using sentences that include the word YOU! *"You should floss more because," "You are making it hard on yourself by not getting the treatment," "You should spend some money on your teeth."* You message will ruin any chances you may have for developing trust and effective communication.

OTHER HELPFUL SUGGESTIONS THAT SHOULD IMPROVE YOUR CHANCES FOR EFFECTIVE COMMUNICATION:

1. Touch patients gently on the shoulder to show empathy.
2. Use mouthwash.
3. Tell co-workers how much you appreciate them.
4. Thank patients for keeping their appointments.
5. Distribute literature to patients (highlight specific areas of concern, use videos).
6. Smile.
7. Compliment patients on their hygiene; never criticize!
8. Learn one "clean" joke/day.
9. Greet patients with a handshake.
10. Restore your mouth ideally and esthetically (call me and I will personally fix you up with all of the veneers that you need - at cost).

11. Be modest.

NEVER:

1. Criticize the work of other dentists. Never!
2. Lose control or show bad emotions.
3. Be a clown.
4. Complain.
5. Use profanity.
6. Be informal.

EVERY QUALITY, THRIVING DENTAL PRACTICE HAS A DENTIST WITH A GOAL-ORIENTED ATTITUDE, SUPERB PEOPLE SKILLS, AND GREAT COMMUNICATION ABILITIES

YOU CAN'T BECOME SOMEONE UNTIL YOU KNOW WHO YOU ARE

ASK OTHERS HOW THEY FEEL ABOUT YOU

CHANGE IS SOMETIMES MANDATORY

WITHOUT CHANGE YOU CANNOT IMPROVE

CHAPTER 14
THE INITIAL PATIENT APPOINTMENT

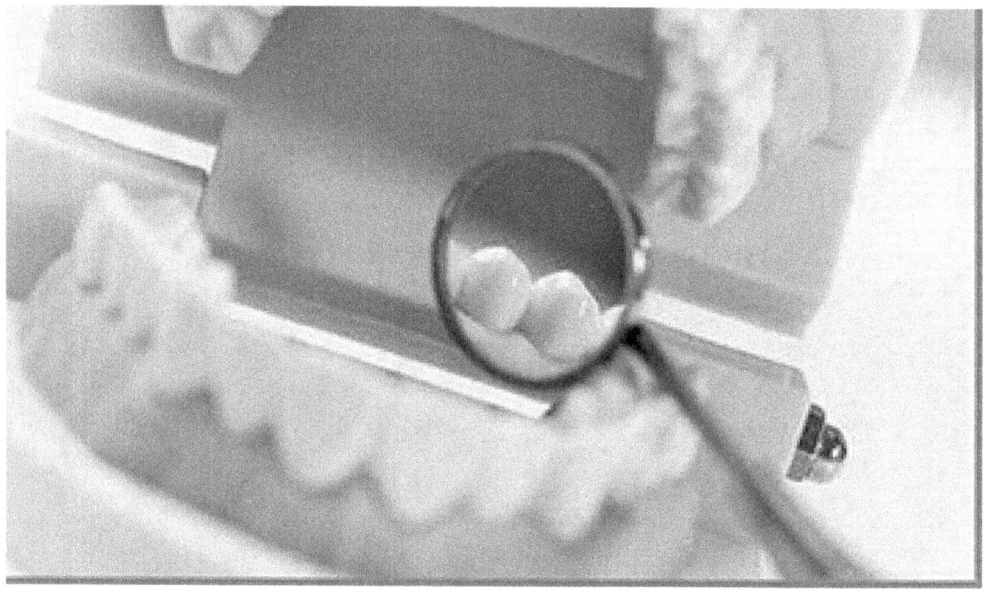

One of the most important parts of your clinical proficiency will be to conduct and complete a thorough initial patient exam. Once this exam is concluded your communication expertise must be called upon to help educate and inform the patient of their needs, in order to motivate them into accepting the recommended treatment. The initial patient appointment should never be hurried and must allow ample time for documentation, education, and relationship building. During the early stages of your career you should never hurry! Allow yourself plenty of time to not only diagnose patient needs but also to help yourself learn and become better at performing a complete exam.

No matter where you end up working, you should insist on adequate and complete dental/medical forms and questionnaires. See the appendix for more details. These forms should include everything from name and address to the following subjects:

1. What name does patient want to be called?
2. Employer name, address, and telephone?
3. Social security #, birthdate, email, work and cell phone numbers.
4. Complete medical history.
5. Past hospitalizations and complications.

6. Name of physician.
7. Allergies.
8. Medications.
9. Past dental history (including questions relating to TMJ, perio treatments, length of time since last appointment, and main concerns)
10. Financial responsibility.
11. Consent to treatment.
12. Likes and dislikes about dentistry.
13. Emergency contact.
14. Signature.

A complete patient exam begins with proper documentation. The patient questionnaire should advise you in regard to their previous medical and dental history and give you information that is necessary to complete their billing and financial responsibilities. The consent should always be explained to the patient by you, the doctor, prior to commencing any treatment.

I always take time to review each patient chart before entering the room. It is nice to familiarize yourself with the patient's past history before you begin your professional relationship. It would be detrimental to your ego for a patient to say "Gee, Doc, I wrote the answers to all of these questions on your sheet!" Re-emphasize the patient history but never sound misinformed, especially after the patient took the time to fill out your forms. It is wise to be prepared for your patient by educating yourself beforehand. This makes people feel special and makes you seem like a caring, thoughtful professional.

All of my initial adult patient exams are scheduled for 40 minutes. During this time the following takes place:

1. Assistant seats patient and records (in writing, in the patient chart) the reason for visit, along with any other patient statements, complaints, and mentions.
2. Doctor is introduced by assistant to patient. Doctor sits in front of patient after personal handshake introduction. Doctor maintains close eye-level contact with patient and asks the following question "Mr. Smith, what concerns you regarding your dental health and what would you like us to accomplish for you?" Other suggested phrases: "Are you happy with your teeth?" or "On a scale of 1 to 10, how would you rate your teeth?"
3. Doctor orders X-rays and study models (if necessary).
4. Doctor review X-rays and begins complete head, neck, and oral exam.
5. Doctor completes treatment plan and patient education.

This fairly simple process is the backbone of your clinical success. Without the right gear you cannot climb the Himalayas; without a complete exam you cannot educate your patients in terms of their dental needs. Without this education you cannot schedule the next appointment. Most of your patients do not see or perceive the need for a majority of the dental work that they may need to have performed. It is up to you to build your patient's confidence, educate them, get their trust, and build the value for the dental work. Again, effective communication must take place.

THE ORAL EXAM

Have you ever seen the "Tacoma Bridge Falls" tape in your high school physics class? If so, then you know that without adequate blue plans and planning you cannot proceed with restorations and oral rehabilitation for your patients. The oral exam is your blueprint to success. The periodic oral exam is the maintenance of your building.

I begin all of my exams with an overall evaluation of the patient. An overall "look" at their physical condition can tell you a lot about your patient.

Do they look like a healthy person?
Is their sking tone healthy?
Are their eyes white or bloodshot or yellow?
Do they breathe easily?
Do their nailbeds look oxygenated?
Are their nails trimmed?
Is their hair groomed and trimmed?
Is their clothing clean?
Do they have body odor?
Are their shoes in good shape?
Are their socks clean?
Is there any ear wax around the ears?
Are their lips chapped?

You do not have to be a medical doctor to gather some insight about a person's overall health. You just need to look and pay attention!

The Dental Exam always starts with a thorough evaluation of the x-rays. I always insist that my assistants are thoroughly trained in taking exceptional x-rays. If the x-rays are lacking I always help the assistant complete the series that I need and make time to teach her how to improve the quality of the x-rays. My exam begins with an overall view of the full mouth series. I check for abnormalities and try to see the forest from the trees before I rev up the chain saw. I have become so proficient at beginning my treatment plans with the aid of x-rays that I can accomplish many diagnostics before picking up the mirror, explorer, and probe. Obviously, the first thing I look for is the picture of the forest with the trees included.

Once my x-ray evaluation is completed I begin my head, neck, and oral exam. This usually starts with an examination of the TMJ area. I palpate the joints for tenderness, and have the patient open a few times to see the ease of mobility. If the patient cannot open more than three finger's width apart, or they complain of sore areas within the musculature, I slow down and evaluate the TMJ a little closer. This usually consists of palpating all of the muscles of mastication and assessing their tenderness. If I detect any pain in the masseters or medial pterygoids upon palpation, I am more than 99.9 % certain that the patient will be undergoing TMJ splint therapy before any other treatment is begun. Patients that grind, brux, and/or clench will present you with many difficulties. Some of the problems will be detailed in chapter 35.

Always ask the patient about any recent or past history of headaches. If the patient has a history or recent chronic problems with headaches/migraines I know that I will take a step back and realize that I will defer any restorative type treatment until we can address the TMJ problem. TMJ/Headache patients will cause most of your clinical problems. If the patient has a history of headaches yet they have no obvious clinical signs of TMJ problems (popping and clicking or crepitus) I will start a deeper investigation into the TMJ problem. This will normally include CT Scans or MRI of their joints. Chronic headache patients are actual TMJ patients who have no clinical symptoms of TMJ problems. Delay their restorative needs until you get a better understanding of their TMJ issues. Visit my website for more info: www.migraineheadachepain.com The information contained on this website will change how your practice dentistry and make your clinical life a thousand times easier once your understand how to diagnose a subclinical TMJ patient.

Next, I will check the occlusion, paying close attention to wear facets, abnormal enamel loss, and potential cusp fractures. I always document the Occlusal Type, as well as any crowding. Collapsed bites are my main concern as they are the leading cause of TMJ and Headaches and dental work that just never seems to fit right. I know that any future restorative work will be largely affected by the occlusal harmony. Furthermore, TMJ patients will require occlusal rehabilitation often involving orthodontics or prosthodontic reconstruction. Trying to fit partials and crowns on patients with collapsed occlusion is like trying to paddle upstream.. Most of your dental work will be based on a balanced occlusal scheme.

Learn to evaluate the vertical dimensions of occlusion and take your time in assessing the patient's occlusion.

Once the TMJ has been examined, I begin an evaluation of the head and neck area. I palpate all lymph nodes and other areas of the facial region. Your dental school instructors have spend plenty of time with you on this important part. Refer back to that education.

The teeth are finally examined for caries, mobility, wear, abrasion, erosion, and attrition. My final job is to complete a periodontal screening, which usually consists of a probation of the pocket depths. At this time I always re-check my x-rays to make sure that I have documented all interproximal calculus deposits, as well as bone loss, and furcation involvements.

Next, I look for missing teeth, infections, impactions, unrestorable teeth, bone loss, hypererupted teeth, abnormalities, etc. Review your dental school basics and follow them!

The bitewings are my most important shots. I sometimes take three per side, especially if there are any rotated teeth and the contacts need different views in order to "break open." The bitewings help me accomplish my caries documentation, as well as periodontal evaluation and occlusal analysis. Vertical BWs may also be necessary if there is more than 40% bone loss. You want to see where the horizontal bone level is and whether you have decay on the roots. **I always analyze my bitewings for decay, bone level, abnormal occlusal loads on bone, furcation involvements, hypereruptions, thickness of enamel, abnormal wear, poor margins, open contacts, root canals without crowns, etc.**

Train your eye to pick up infrabony and vertical bone loss because these findings usually indicate hard to diagnose periodontal problems, as well as uneven occlusal loads.

Once I am finished, I double-check my chart entries and make sure that all records are completely documented. I always try to complete as much of the fact gathering effort in the same room where the patient is seated. Taking the time to review x-rays, and intra-oral photos, shows your patient that you are being careful and not hurrying. Finally, I begin my case presentation to my patient. If I do not have the adequate time to get to know my patient, or if I need to evaluate mounted study models, I always reschedule my patient. I like to have time to complete my exam and finalize my treatment plan.

Do not be in a hurry to present a treatment plan to a patient, especially if there is a lot of work involved. If you have any doubts or questions, especially about the occlusion, wait until you have had time to thoroughly complete your evaluation.

MEASURE SUCCESS BY HOW FAR YOUR TALENTS CAN TAKE YOU

CHAPTER 15
THE PATIENT CASE PRESENTATION (YOU NEVER GET A SECOND CHANCE TO MAKE A FIRST IMPRESSION)

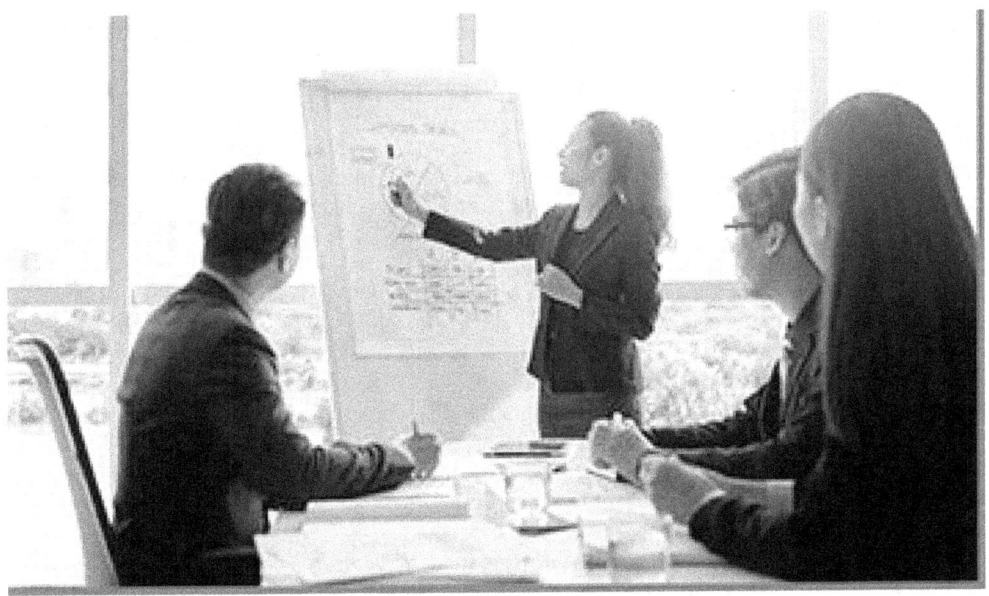

I live by the basic philosophy that I cannot be everything to everyone. That is why I make my case presentations according to my practice philosophy. This philosophy includes ideal dentistry and respect for myself and my profession. I always present a patient's entire dental needs in accordance with the best possible dental care available. This never takes into account the patient's financial or mental condition. Patients are never afraid to tell you that they cannot afford a $4000 round-house bridge or six lower implants. But I am also never afraid to present these options to all of my patient's according to their needs. It takes a lot of sales calls to get an order...it takes a lot of case presentations to "sell" the big-ticket items. Don't ever be afraid to present optimal dentistry.

It may take 10 crown explanations to get one crown procedure. It may take 100 bridge presentations to get one patient commitment. The odds are still in your favor as long as you keep educating. Do not ever pre-judge people. I have sold $15000 bridges to patients wearing $2 Salvation Army clothing..

Present optimal dentistry to all of your patients, unless they clearly inform you that they are not interested in their oral health.

Your case presentation relies upon your knowledge of dentistry. It also relies upon your information of the drawbacks and complications of treatment. You must always present and inform. Your first few minutes of contact with a new patient is more crucial than any other time. It will determine whether you will build a trusting relationship, or whether the new patient will visit another office. Your goal during this period is to portray self-confidence, creativity, empathy, and consideration. You must know what you are talking about and inform your patient about their needs in a confident manner. This confidence builds trust and gains case acceptance.

You must also be creative because dentistry is a multi-discipline approach. Patients want you to talk their language, not dental jargon. Obviously, you have to show empathy and consideration for their desires. This is effectively done through the active practice of listening. If you feel that your communication and listening skills are not adequate, audio-tape yourself during some new patient case presentations and evaluate yourself from an outside perspective. Better yet, get some input from your staff.

Patients come to you because they have a need. They want something done and they will buy it if they like the person selling it. Although they usually do not know much about their particular dental needs, they have sought you and your office because they believe that they have a need. It is up to you to diagnose their need and gain treatment acceptance through effective communication. Without building trust through effective communication you have no chance of fulfilling the patient's need. 99% of the time you know the reason for the patient's visit. You must always address the patient's concern, first. You can inform them about their other needs after you have started discussing what the patient thinks that they need done, first and foremost.

"Mr. Patient, I understand that you are having some discomfort with the tooth on this side. Please tell me more about your problem."

"Mrs. Patient, I understand that your gums are bleeding when you brush. Can you tell me what else concerns you?"

"Mr. Patient, I understand that you are concerned about getting cavities. Can you tell me why you believe that you are getting cavities?"

"Mrs. Patient, I understand that you are here for a general check-up. Is there anything that concerns you regarding your teeth?"

"Mr. Patient, I understand that you are not very happy with your teeth and you would like us to see what can be done to improve your mouth."

Whatever choice of words you make, you must remember that you have to take into consideration the perceived needs of your patient before addressing any oral findings. Address their perceived need to start with. Develop a relationship, and then worry about optimal dental health. Do not start discussing your treatment plan until you get to know your patient and you have had time to build trust. <u>Address their perceived need, first and foremost.</u> Then continue with your findings.

Once you begin a case presentation, and you have broken the ice with the new patient, you have to make them aware of the possible dental care that you can offer. **More importantly, you must always cover the consequences of non-treatment.** There are usually many more negative aspects of delaying treatment than there are complications of receiving the treatment. Use this sentence to educate them about their main concerns and their other dental needs:

"Mr. Smith, your tooth needs _____, because_____. If you elect not to have this procedure done, then the following consequences will happen _____."

Again: **YOU NEED, BECAUSE!**

One of the most powerful words in the English dictionary: B-E-C-A-U-S-E!!!

Do not consider this to be negative advertising. It is your job to explain the negative aspects of delaying treatment to all of your patients. Some will understand your educative purpose, others will simply not care. Do not allow your dead-beat patients to slow you down from presenting optimal dental care to all of your patrons. Remember: all people want to attain pleasure and avoid pain!!!

Dentistry has always been shadowed by the inability to make the patient realize the importance of the need for their dental treatment. This has usually been a result of a lack of our ability to show this need to our patients. This has changed in recent years. At my office I have an intraoral camera. Practitioners who do not own this technology are living in the dark ages. Your patients are used to making purchasing decisions by seeing and feeling. An intra-oral camera will help them visualize their needs, just like a dressing room at the local department store allows them to see the new clothes that they are about to purchase. If you are going to be using a camera during your first years in practice, follow these basics:

a. Show patients their failing amalgams. Explain the "separation" of filling from tooth, along with any noticeable fractures and discolorations, which indicate recurrent decay.

b. Note large amalgams and/or composites. Concentrate your case presentation on these time-bomb teeth. The fracture chances of an MOD amalgam/composite with less than 50% cuspal anatomy is high. Inform patients of these potential problems. When a patient fractures a tooth that you fore-warned them about (even if it happens 5 years later) your credibility will sky-rocket.

c. Show bleeding gums and tartar build-up. Don't be afraid to probe the gums to elicit suppuration).

d. Show gross caries, infections, etc.

e. Provide the patient with a photo of the important findings.

f. Save photos for insurance processing. Save photos for legal documentation: capture lesions, normalities, abnormalities, existing fillings, cracks, and other problems that cannot be documented with x-rays and charting.

Other helpful ideas for using an intraoral camera:

1. Use Invisalign's QR code so patients can do a before/after simulation. Helps to sell a lot more cosmetic work than Invisalign cases.

2. Use the camera to check for decay, crown margin finish, or other areas where you may need magnification.

3. Take pre-op and post-op photos, especially when doing cosmetics (even on posterior teeth).

4. Show healthy areas of the mouth, and quality dental care, so that patients can see the differences between this and needed work.

Most dentists that use an intraoral camera perform a variety of cosmetic procedures. The intraoral camera is a great adjunct to helping you sell cosmetic dentistry. A helpful phrase that you should use is as follows: *"Mr. Smith, on a scale of 1 to 10 how would you rate the appearance of your teeth?"* Use the camera to help the patient realize how that rating can be improved and how their life can benefit from this improvement.

The intraoral camera is a great aid in helping you achieve case acceptance and improving your communication. Your patients are going to present you with four obstacles that prevent them from to undergoing dental treatment. Again, at the sake of being redundant, these factors are:

1. **FEAR (an emotional and psychological factor).**
2. **MONEY**
3. **TIME AWAY FROM WORK**
4. **OUTCOME OF TREATMENT (esthetics, comfort, longevity, etc.)**

You must refer to these obstacles during your presentation, and at all other times. Every patient will exhibit at least one of these obstacles. Sometimes they will tell you exactly which one. Sometimes you may have to ask. But you must develop your presentation around these barriers.

The following section will provide you with some communication examples to help you improve your presentation skills and achieve better case acceptance. Adapt these ideas as best fitted for your individual personality. You must realize that the patient does not think like you do and usually knows very little about dentistry.

What the patient thinks they need, what the patient wants, and what the patient actually needs can be very different.

You must uncover and discover the patient's needs through effective communication and presentation. The most important factors in communicating with your patients are the patient's level of desire, the complexity of the case, and the patient's level of understanding.

Your goal is to motivate patients to accept their needed treatment. You must develop trust because 99% of your patients make choices based on emotions and trust. When it comes to motivating your patients to accept their treatment plan your technical skills are not as important as your ability to perform the art of listening and communicating.

To overcome the first and most important obstacle -FEAR - please refer to chapter 21. You must learn how to educate and inform your patients about your ability to prevent pain and discomfort. You must take the time to explain this to your patients. Otherwise, you cannot proceed to overcome the other obstacles and present your treatment plan. You can read chapter 21 now, and come back to the following sections.

Most of your patients will present you with financial difficulties. All case presentations lead to discussion of cost. It is your responsibility to build value for the needed dental treatment by communicating the advantages and disadvantages of treatment. Most patients will value the cost of their required treatment once they realize the consequences of delaying their needs because all people want to avoid pain and problems.

How do you overcome objections to cost?

The petty, cheezy response: "Mr. Smith, that procedure costs so much because I have high overhead in my office and the lab bill is enormous. With rent and employees and taxes, etc. it costs me $100 per hour just to reserve this chair for you."

The cerebral alternative:

Consider that case acceptance hinges on patient trust: to gain this trust, you must build confidence. This may be difficult with new patients.. This may or may not be true with patients of record. In either case, follow these simple solutions for overcoming fee issues and helping patients see the positive outcomes of treatment:

1. Evaluate your fees and make sure that you are in the "ball-park" with the customary and usual fees for your area. New patients will price-shop. The same customers that drive 20 miles to save $10 on a pair of Nikes will be the same patients questioning your fees.
2. Spend a minimum of 40 minutes with new patients performing their exam, X-rays, and education. Do not hurry, hustle, or appear rushed to new patients, even if it is only a consultation appointment. Build trust through a professional introduction, a thorough medical history, good eye contact, listening, and having a friendly bedside manner.
3. Gather all necessary information during the patient examination appointment. An intraoral camera is your second right hand!

4. Once you have finalized a treatment plan, discuss the patient's needs and the consequences of delaying or denying the necessary treatment.
5. Discuss insurance benefits and/or financial arrangements.
6. Never discuss your costs and problems. This is a guaranteed way to lose the trust of your patients!

Never diagnose a patient's wants, needs, desires, or pocketbook. Present optimal treatment at all times!!!

If you focus on the patient's needs and the benefits of treatment you can overcome many obstacles. Of course you may present cost saving alternatives (if they are possible) as long as you also explain the drawbacks and possible problems that may occur if the patient chooses these options. It is wise to have the patient sign their record to indicate that they chose the less than optimal procedure.

All patients want to avoid PAIN AND PROBLEMS! People do something because of either fear or pleasure. Center your conversation and sales skills on making the patient aware of how the treatment will prevent:

1. **future pain**
2. **future cost**
3. **future problems**

Explain to them how they will benefit from the treatment and how they will receive pleasure out of the treatment.

CROWNS:

In order to be a profitable dentist you must learn to treatment plan crowns and bridges. Too often, dentists fail to recommend the necessary crown treatment. If a tooth has less than 50% cuspal coverage (i.e. has MODBXYZ amalgam) it needs to be crowned, even if that amalgam has great anatomy. It may also needs to be endodontically treated, unless you are certain that the pulp is unaffected. I tell all of my patients with such teeth the following:

"Mr. Smith, this tooth with the large filling has decay along with hundreds of small fractures...cracks like you would see in your driveway. You can see many of these cracks on this intraoral picture. One day soon, you will bite on your favorite food and the tooth could break completely. If it breaks deep into the root we will have to remove it. I am recommending a crown to protect it and prevent you from losing it. During the process of fabricating the crown it is possible that the pulp of the tooth could be damaged. Therefore, it may be necessary to perform a root canal and core, in order to prevent your tooth from getting infected."

You must explain why the cost is so high:
- It is an investment for your health and your mouth.
- It will prevent pain because the tooth will not crack any more.

- It will prevent you from any future expenses.
- It will restore your ability to chew, smile and speak.
- It will prevent the loss of the tooth. If you lose it, other teeth will shift position in the mouth and eventually cause you to lose many other teeth, which of course will become even more expensive to repair/replace.
- A crown is your best alternative because it is custom-made to fit your tooth in our laboratory. It takes approximately one hour to prepare the tooth for the laboratory. We use over 100 different steps to adjust the tooth properly during this first appointment. It takes 5 days to fabricate the crown in the laboratory, and then another 30 minutes to seat the crown on your tooth, at your second appointment. Many state-of-the art materials are used to accurately fit your crown. The crown will last you a lifetime, with proper care.

Obviously your treatment plans will include many other treatment needs and procedures. The following list may help overcome some of the obstacles for other common patient needs:

PERIO:

"Mr. Smith, I know that the cost of this treatment is important, but consider what will happen if you decide to delay. You will not have the option of rebuilding your teeth once they are lost. When you lose these teeth you will need dentures and you will be very unhappy because your jaws will shrink, your smile will be affected, and your general health will suffer."

DENTURES:

"Mr. Smith, your denture choices are as follows: you have the option of choosing a cost-saving economy denture at $___, or you have the option of choosing a regular denture at $___, or the option of choosing our deluxe denture at $___. The only difference between the dentures is the cost of the material that is used to make the dentures. Obviously, the deluxe dentures will last you longer than the economy dentures because the material is of much higher quality. We use high-impact acrylic and the most naturally looking teeth available on the market. The regular denture is the <u>same</u> as our deluxe denture except that it does not include a soft liner cushion which makes the dentures feel like pillows on your gums. All of our dentures are custom made to fit your mouth as perfectly and comfortably as possible. Remember that you will use your teeth for many hours each day and you want to feel good, look good, and chew well."

(author's note: at our office we have 3 different sets of dentures that we offer patients...we price our economy set at $695, our regular set at $950, and our deluxe at $1400. The deluxe includes soft liners and clear palates if the patient requests them. The $695 dentures bring many price shoppers to our office through effective advertising. I have yet to fabricate a $695 denture. Once patients realize the benefit of the regular or deluxe denture they always opt for them. If you ever have to fabricate an economy denture I'm sure that your lab can accommodate you)

FILLINGS

"Mr. Smith, I have shown you these cavities on your x-rays and in your mouth. The cost of these fillings is minimal if you consider what will happen if you delay treatment. Once these cavities get larger and/or the teeth start breaking, the cost of root canals with build-ups and crowns will be a lot higher. Maybe even ten times more. This does not even take into consideration the number of extra appointments it will take to salvage these teeth at that time. Of course, you also have to consider the possible pain and discomfort you will experience if these teeth get infected or broken."

COSMETICS

"Mrs. Smith, I can assure you that this work will do more to enhance your natural beauty than other cosmetics. It will increase your confidence and self-esteem. The most important benefit will be the fact that you will look much younger and much more beautiful when the work is completed!"

(author's note: at my office I do mock-up bonding for all possible cosmetic work. Glidewell Laboratories has a great video-tape on this procedure. It involves using composite, without etching or bonding. This is detailed in Chapter 38. You simply mold the composite on the teeth just as though you were doing it as a restorative procedure, without actually bonding the composite. You dry the teeth, place the composite, mold it with a brush or plastic instrument, and let the patient see it in their mouth. I like to take photos of the mock-up and send the photo home with the patient. You should not cure the composite. It will stay on the teeth long enough to give the patient the time to see the improvement. Watch your cosmetic sales double when you use this technique.

ROOT CANALS

"Mr. Smith, a root canal is the last line of defense for saving a troubled tooth. Most of the time it is 99.99% successful, if you follow our recommendations. If you decide to take the tooth out it will be much more expensive to replace the tooth with bridges or implants. A missing tooth will cause other problems because your teeth will shift out of their normal alignment. This mis-alignment will place stress on your jaws and your muscles, thereby preventing you from chewing, speaking, and smiling properly. Eventually, a lot more of your teeth will drift, like dominoes, and your problems will worsen. Even low-cost partials will be more expensive because they have to be replaced every 5 years. Your small investment now will be an immediate benefit for your mouth because it will prevent future problems and more expenses."

REPLACEMENT PARTIALS

"Mr. Smith, replacing your partials every 5 years, and relining them every 12 months, is a minimal investment that you have to make to keep your teeth in proper alignment and prevent your jaws from not being balanced. Improperly fitting partials (which happens when your gums and bone shrink under the fake teeth) place a lot of stress on your remaining teeth. This stress can cause you to possibly lose them. Once you lose your remaining teeth the only alternative will be full dentures. As you know, dentures are not as easy to wear as partials and you will have a problem tasting and chewing your favorite foods."

SEALANTS

"Mrs. Smith, little Johnny just got his 6 year molars in. Most kids develop cavities on these teeth by the time they are 12 years old. We can place sealants on each of his molars now at the cost of $____ or you can take the chance and wait to pay $____ if he gets those cavities. The sealants are like wax for your car. They will protect his teeth against cavities on the top of the tooth as long as he brushes and flosses properly. Brushing and flossing, alone, may not prevent these cavities. There are no shots and drills involved."

Finally, use the following sentence for all patients:
"Mr. Patient, would you like to discuss any reason that may prevent you from having this procedure done?"

- THINK LIKE A CONSUMER
- TALK LIKE A CONSUMER
- ACT LIKE A CONSUMER!!!!!!!!!!!!!!!!!!!!!!!!!!!!!

PATIENTS BUY YOUR TREATMENT PLAN BECAUSE THEY

- LIKE YOU
- TRUST YOU
- RESPECT YOU!!!!!!!!!!!!!!!!!!!

During your case presentations you must get into the habit of using colorful brochures to help explain the patient's needs. This is very important with the "analytical" patients. The more visual aids you use, the more you increase your percentage of acceptance. A picture is worth a thousand words!!! Always highlight key points in the brochure and draw your own pictures if necessary. Let the patient take the brochures home and insist that they call you with any questions.

In order to overcome the last obstacle -TIME - you do not need to jump through hoops. Expand your schedule and make yourself available to your patients! Emphasize the importance of scheduled appointments to your patients at all times. Take the time, personally, to explain to your patients how important it is for them to keep their scheduled appointment: *"Mr. Patient, I am going to go to the front desk and make sure that I can RESERVE the necessary time to complete your treatment...when it is convenient for you."*

Patients break appointments for various reasons, but the most common cause of failed appointments is due to lack of communication and failure to overcome the three obstacles on your part.

Once you have hurdled these barriers stress the importance of keeping appointments.

Remember, patients are not able to evaluate your clinical expertise. Sure, they may have heard that you are a great dentist, but many patients are usually wrong about their previous dentist and about the type of dental work that they may have received elsewhere.

People think about the dentist and refer other patients if you did not hurt them, did not charge them a lot of money, and gave them a convenient appointment.

Many times you may even have to answer the following patient question: "Why didn't my previous dentist tell me about these problems?" Of course, the patient may be thinking about whether you are trying to sell them something. As long as you have taken the time to gather data, communicate the needs to the patient, and show them those needs, you have done your job. Trust has been developed and your patient will be motivated to meet their needs.

SUPERIOR SERVICE IS ALWAYS THE FIRST AND LAST THING THAT A CUSTOMER REMEMBERS

SUCCESS IN BUSINESS AND PATIENT SERVICE GO HAND IN HAND

CHAPTER 16
TREATMENT PLANNING

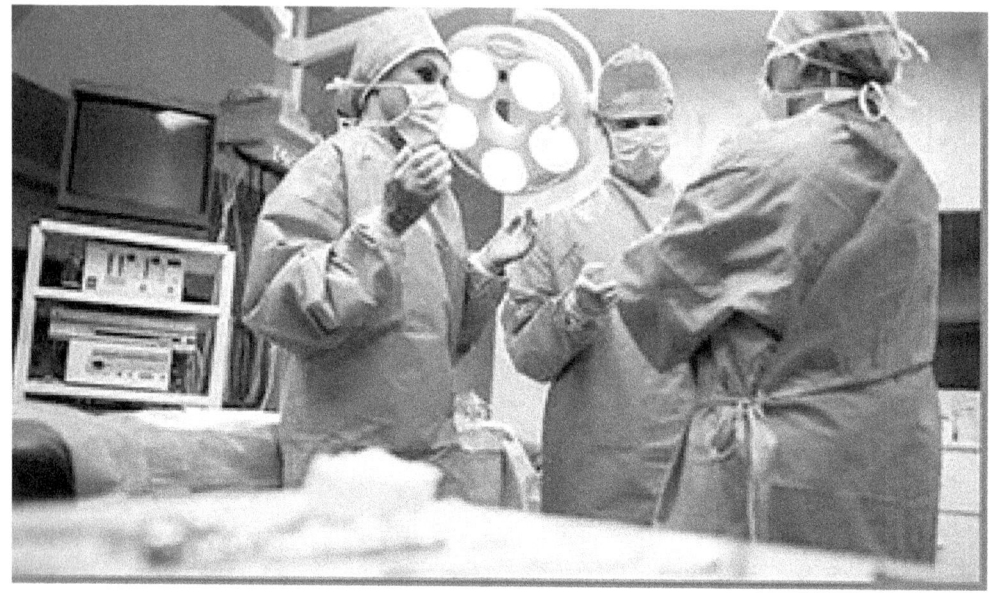

Have you ever gone shopping in a store that had no price tags? What would you feel like walking up to the counter and hearing "Mr. Smith, that will be $2199 for those jeans and t- shirts!"? Does the word 'overwhelmed' come to mind?

Patients should always receive a written treatment plan. Consider it your store's price tag. Whether or not your patient has insurance coverage is meaningless. **Everyone must receive a written treatment plan.** Now and then you will perform work on a patient with good insurance coverage. That patient may just be losing their coverage and getting laid off. How would you explain to the patient that they owe you hundreds of dollars not covered by insurance? Take the time to communicate case presentations and discuss treatment plans with all of your patients. The more treatment plans you complete, the better you will become at optimizing them.

All of my treatment plans are entered into the computer. Breakdowns are computed between estimated insurance and patient responsibility. Appointment scheduling is coordinated with the treatment plan. I try to offer cost-saving alternatives to my patients as a secondary treatment option. However, I always present and plan optimal treatment.

For patients with cash payment options, or poor insurance coverage, I try to coordinate scheduling of treatment according to their ability to pay. I never "run" a patient's bill. The ocean was made one drop at a time, and some of your patients will also need to be treated one step at a time. I have many patients who need thousands of dollars of dental work but can only afford to pay $90 a month. Guess how long it takes to complete their work?! I am not a bank and I don't know of any dentist in this country that owns a savings and loan institution. If a patient with limited finances does not return to my office because I will not complete a $3000 bridge for $90 monthly payments, I sleep well at night. There is some other chump who is going to pay to perform this patient's work. I don't want it to be me!!!

When a patient does not present with financial barriers and/or they have great dental insurance coverage, I treatment plan my dental work by quadrant philosophy. This is very simple: if I am going to numb the lower right mandibular quadrant, that patient will have optimal treatment finished in the entire quadrant. All old amalgams will be replaced, all root canals will be completed, and all other restorative work finished. Of course, the periodontal condition must be healthy! If periodontal scaling or surgery is planned, this is completed before any work (except palliative) is commenced. I do not perform any restorative work on a patient with even the slightest amount of bleeding. It is frustrating and non-profitable dentistry. The periodontal condition must be sound and healthy!!!

I also try to expand quadrant dentistry to include multiple quadrant dentistry. I limit my appointments to less than 3 hours. Whatever the patient can tolerate during this time, I will complete. The only limitation is patient compliance and 10 carpules of anesthetic.

Upper and lower quadrants on one side are usually completed in one seating. This is the most profitable way to accomplish your dental work. Your patients will also appreciate the fact that they do not have to schedule multiple appointments. The faster you can finish a patient's treatment, the more appreciative they will be. Just make sure that the patient has approved your quadrant treatment sequence and there are not medical contraindications.

The major roadblock you will encounter during optimal treatment planning is trying to decide exactly what the patient will have done and what will happen to certain teeth. Will that deep caries be a root canal, core, crown? Or will it be an MOD composite? Can periodontal surgery save all the teeth in the lower right quadrant or do we need to plan for implants? My basic suggestion to you is to always plan for the worst. I tell all of my patients that their treatment plan includes the worst possible scenario: *"Mrs. Patient, this written treatment plan contains all of the estimates for the problems we talked about. I have detailed the best possible dental care and taken into account all of the possible alternatives and complications. If we can perform the least costly alternative, we will do so. However, I cannot tell you what is going to happen with the following teeth _____ until we start the actual treatment."* Do not ever be afraid to overdiagnose. This does not mean overtreat!

At the sake of being redundant, get in the habit of doing the following for your patients:

1. Study their completed medical/dental histories.
2. Take the time to get to know the patient and their personalities.
3. Develop a professional relationship based on trust.
4. Present optimal treatment.
5. Complete written treatment plans for all patients.
6. Attempt to perform quadrant dentistry.

7. Never fall into the belief that increase patient flow leads to increased income. It is increased case acceptance that leads to increased income. Case acceptance is only possible through effective communication and patient education.

CHAPTER 17
INSURANCE/COLLECTIONS

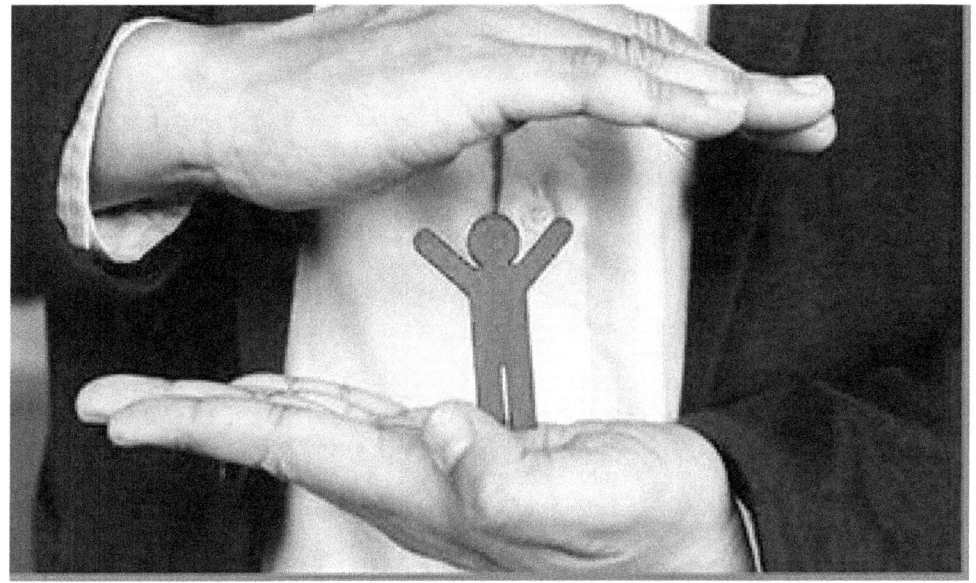

Whether you will be an owner or associate, your paycheck will depend on your ability to perform dentistry and collect the money for your efforts. You must begin to educate yourself on the topic of dental insurance and payments. Your treatment plans, and eventual completion of procedures, will depend on coordination of third party benefits and patient finances. You cannot jump into performing dental care to patients without considering your patient's ability to pay or share in the cost of treatment.

The full cost of treatment must be quoted before, not after, treatment has begun.

Sending statements for services not discussed is a sure way to upset your patients. You must learn to coordinate insurance benefits as much as you must improve your communication skills. Obviously, you must also realize that you should be more concerned with what your patients value for their mouths, and are willing to spend, instead of what the insurance company will pay.

Dental insurance carriers are merely intermediaries that act as fiduciaries in distributing funds between labor and management. The money that is paid out is directly tied to your patient's paychecks. Obviously the carriers make money by holding and investing the funds while attempting not to pay out. It's sort of like a rigged slot machine. Despite this cynical view, it is important to remember that the type and amount of benefits available depends on the contractual

119

agreements between the insurance company and labor management. It is your responsibility to find out what the benefits and exclusions may be.

Insurance companies are governed by the IRS and Department of Labor via the ERISA (Employee Retirement Income Security) Act of 1974. Basically, ERISA requires each carrier to specifically cite the reason for any benefit denial. The carrier must cite specific references to the plan's provisions which justify any denial of a benefit. The review procedure must also be outlined.

At the same time, the FTC acts as a policeman against us dentists. It limits our ability to gather and set fees, or do anything that is considered a threat to free competition. As a dentist you are not allowed, by law, to call another dentist down the street and ask about his/her prices. This is considered a violation of free enterprise and competition. Our dental organizations are also prohibited from coercing or entering into agreements with insurance companies to alter provisions of dental plans.

As a rule dental insurance plans do not pay the entire cost of dental care. Most programs include many provisions to limit the amount of covered services.

Dental insurance is offered to REDUCE the cost of dental care, NOT to ELIMINATE it.

- In 1958 dental coverage provided patients with $1000 worth of benefits per calendar year.
- In 1997 most dental coverage provided patients with only $1000 of benefits per calendar year yet $1000 depreciated to $200 since 1958
- In 2020, we are lucky to see plans that have $2000 coverage
- From 1997 to 2020, $1000 has depreciated to $400

What a joke, heh!?

The most common insurance programs are as follows:

1. Fee For Service Programs

Most widely used insurance programs where the dentist is paid his usual fees, provided that the fees are not in excess of the fees charged by the other dentists in the area. Normally the doctor is not asked to participate with these programs and payment is made directly to the doctor, as long as the patient has authorized this direct payment. The patient is responsible for all fees, irrespective of what the insurance covers. Normally, these insurance programs have deductibles.

At my office we try not to bill the patient for the difference between our fees and remittance fees unless the discrepancy is larger than 5 % of the fees. Co-payments, of course, must be adhered to at all times. All insurance carriers insists that the patient is charged their co-payment at the time of services.

Programs, such as Blue Cross and Delta, are considered fee for service plans, however you must participate with them in order to be able to get direct payment. Also, these carriers, will only pay and allow certain amounts and you cannot bill the patient for the difference. Even co-payments must be calculated according to the maximum allowable by the carrier. Sometimes you are not allowed to bill the patient for services that the carrier does not cover (i.e. a periodontal cleaning within 90 days of periodontal treatment).

2. Scheduled Fee Programs

Such programs pay the doctor a fixed fee for services, as determined by the carrier. Normally these fees are less than 50% of normal fees. The patient must provide you with a booklet of the fees, or the carrier must send a list of the fees before definite financial estimates and treatment plans can be completed. Government sponsored programs (i.e. Social Services) fall under this category, however you cannot charge the patient the difference in fees (Medicaid allows a certain amount and only pays a certain amount - usually, in the form of peanuts). All other scheduled fee programs usually involve patient payment responsibility, according to what the carrier will not cover. Unless you participate with any such plans, you can charge the patient the entire difference between the fee that the carrier will cover and your total fee.

3. Discount Service Programs, PPOs, DMOs, etc.

These programs are similar to fee for service benefit programs, however they involve deductibles and maximums that must be adhered to at all times. You have to sign your life away and be a participating member! As a generalization, they usually allow you to charge about 80% of your fees, as a maximum. The patient co-payment is calculated based on the maximum allowable fee, as dictated by the carrier. You cannot charge the patient more than what is allowed and/or any difference between your full fees and covered fees.

Some of these plans may do nothing more than allow you to charge only certain specified fees to the subscribers. In turn, your name and practice location is listed, free of charge, in their directory. You will get no payment from the company, just free advertising. Insist upon full payment at time of services from these patients, because your fees will be discounted at least 20%, on the average.

4. Capitation Programs

Sign up, receive a certain amount per month per patient times number of total patients, and try not to do too much dental work. Use these programs only if your chairs are empty and you're starving. Consider them during the early part of your career. As an average if you have 100 subscribers, you can receive $1000 per month, whether or not you do any work on these patients. If all of them need root canals and crowns, then try to delay treatment as much as possible and do as little as possible at each appointment. Limit chair time for these patients and use them to promote your business and fill your empty times. Perform no work until patient has paid any possible co-payments, before treatment commences. Educate yourself on capitation programs if you decide to join any of them.

You must begin to educate yourself on dental insurance and prices. Many practitioners are still clueless in regard to optimal insurance coordination and processing. It never ceases to amaze me how many dentists run to full-day seminars attempting to learn about insurance and collections.

Almost all of the necessary information that you will ever need is contained in the manuals supplied by Blue Cross, Delta, Medicaid, and other booklets provided by insurance companies. All you have to do is spend a few days reading this material and getting familiar with the different policies and codes. <u>All of the education that you need is provided in these manuals or in other online sources.</u>

One of the first things you have to consider is becoming a participating provider with insurance carriers such as Delta, Medicaid, Metlife, Guardian, and Blue Cross. Participating status means that you gain the ability to receive checks for dental work performed on patients that have these forms of insurance. If you don't participate, the carriers will reimburse for treatment, but will send the checks directly to the patients. They will also pay at a lower than customary fee schedule. Although I feel that this is unconstitutional, you have no recourse. You must abide and agree if you need these plans.

Once you become a participating provider you must adhere to the requirements and rules set forth by these insurance carriers. Make sure that you know these regulations or you could end up paying thousands of dollars in penalties at a later date (if you are audited). Basically, these companies (i.e. Delta) want you to charge the same fees to cash patients as you do to their company. They also want you to collect co-payment responsibilities and not provide discounts. Of course, they will audit your charts to make sure that all procedures billed for have been provided and noted. Make sure that you keep all x-rays in the charts, document all procedures that have been performed, log in all appropriate dates, and legibly write all pertinent documentation to substantiate treatment and follow-up care. You are at the mercy of these insurance companies. There is no judge and jury if you ever get audited and the auditor deems your records to be lacking or to be inappropriate. They can hang and lynch you without trial.

All other insurance companies do not require participating contracts, except for certain PPOs or managed care programs. You will be bombarded with letters from all of these other carriers in no time at all. All fee for service companies, other than the participating ones, usually require no contracts with you. There are hundred of these companies. They are basically all the same.

Capitation programs are still around but decreasing in number. These carriers require that you sign a contract with them and they will provide you with a consistent method of payment. This is usually in the form of a monthly payment based on the number of patients that they sign up for your office. Reimbursement varies. A simple explanation is as follows: Cap Program signs up 100 subscribers for your office. For every patient they will pay you $10 per month. Whether or not you see these patients, you will receive $1000 per month, each and every month. If one patient comes to the office and requires $2000 worth of work, you must perform it. The patient may or may not be responsible for lab or out-of-pocket costs for some of the treatments. The more work you perform on capitation plans, the more money you lose. The less work you do and the less patients you see, the more you make.

Capitation plans are usually not conducive to quality dental care. Of course this depends on the individual practitioner. In my opinion, they are a prostituted insult to the profession. At the same time they are a necessary evil for some practitioners, especially recent graduates. As you enter the profession you may find yourself providing a lot of services to these patients. Use this drawback to your advantage: market yourself to these patients and their families and friends. In later years you may be surprised how many "good" referrals come from capitation patients. These patients usually have good jobs. They're just poor victims of great marketing put forth by the insurance carriers.

Always take time to educate yourself on dental insurance. Don't sign any agreements before you have done your homework. Once you have completed study of the manuals provided by the carriers you will have a thorough knowledge of insurance reimbursement.

You should begin to memorize the most commonly used insurance codes. <u>I make all of my Routing Slip entries by using codes.</u> Why write out exam, x-rays, Prophy, Fluoride, etc. when I can note codes 110, 210, 1110, and 1201 instead?! It makes it easier on the billing director and it helps to constantly remind you of insurance requirements. This is the simplest way of writing down the procedures performed, without having to do a lot of scribbling. If your office changes insurance billers often then it is also makes it easy to transcribe the codes into a claim without having to look up the code/description every five seconds. It reduces your employee training time. The other important documentation pertains to your chart clinical notes: amount of anesthetic used, medications given, treatment performed, materials used, sequence of steps, complications of treatment, verbal patient statements, etc.

Learn your codes!!!

Your treatment plans must be made in accordance with insurance coverage, when indicated. Your insured patients expect to pay very little out of their pocket for their treatment. You must do everything possible to maximize their benefits and inform your patients, without forgetting to establish value of the dental treatment. Don't ever start treatment until you have finished the case presentation and you have verified eligibility/benefits. Become familiar with the different categories of coverage:

Completion of all relevant insurance information is critical to expediting payment and decreasing headaches. The completion of a claim starts with the collection of data before the patient is ever seen.

The following information must be gathered before calling insurance carrier:

1. **Correctly spelled Last Name, First Name, Middle Name.**
2. **Birth-Date.**
3. **Social Security Number.**
4. **Employer.**
5. **Policy number and group number.**
6. **Patient's address, employer's address, and any contact persons at work.**
7. **Secondary coverage by spouse or other family members.**

The following information must be checked when calling the insurance carrier (whether you are being assisted by computer or representative):

1. **Effective date of insurance and time limits on coverage.**
2. **Type of insurance program.**
3. **Deductible (self and family).**
4. **Annual maximum.**
5. **Renewal date of coverage.**
6. **Exclusions in coverage or exceptions in coverage.**
7. **Coverage breakdown and co-payments (this must include separating different procedures under the different categories of breakdown...i.e. A, B, C) Every contract and insurance carrier could be different in their categorization of procedural separation so it is important to ask the co-payment for procedures. A standard guideline is to separate procedures as follows:**

Category A - exams, cleanings, x-rays, palliative treatments
Category B - restorative, crown and bridge, perio, endo
Category C - dentures, partials, bridges, and possibly crowns
Category D - orthodontics

8. **ask about any secondary coverage that may be listed**

Your office should have an Insurance Form sheet to help assist your front desk in properly obtaining all necessary insurance information. If you do not have such aids please consider ordering our office management program.

Note: x-rays may fall under A or B; <u>crowns can fall under B or C;</u> endodontic or perio treatments may fall under B or C. Double check, always!!!

Missing tooth clause for any contract means that if the patient had any teeth extracted prior to coverage, the insurance will not pay for replacements of these teeth. Be careful with this policy before you treatment plan any bridges or partials.

If your computer is set up correctly and the insurance data is entered properly It is very simple to do a treatment plan with complete co-payment responsibility breakdown. Inform and educate your patient before you surprise them with a bill. You will lose patients if you perform without informing. Don't get in the habit of performing dentistry on patients that tell you they can't afford to pay their responsibility even if this money is less than 15% of the total. You will lose money and get yourself in hot water with the insurance companies. Collect co-payments and inform patients!!!

A QUICK WORD ABOUT DEPENDENTS

Children and young adults under the age of 18 are normally listed under their parents insurance. If the dependent is between the age of 18 and 25 they must have special dependent status (i.e. student) to qualify for coverage.

REGULATIONS:

1. **Waving Co-Pays violates our agreement with carriers.** It cannot be done. If the patient cannot pay their portion then their account must be documented with: *"the patient cannot afford to participate in the cost of treatment at this time"*. You must bill the patient 3 times and if you get no payment then do a Bad Debt Write-Off (BDWO.) All of the statements must be documented in their account.
2. **Discounted fee for treatment:** if giving a discount always bill the discounted fee on the claim. You cannot discount just the co-pay.
3. **Charging non-insurance patients:** make sure that the fee charged to insurance is the same fee charged to non-insurance patients in similar circumstances.
4. **Do not up-code procedures:** example: do not bill surgical extraction instead of a routine extraction if you have not raised a flap and reduced bone.
5. **Accept scheduled fees:** if you are a participating provider and procedure is not covered under plan or patient is out of annual maximum bill scheduled fee instead of your normal fee.

INSURANCE PROCEDURES TO SPEED UP PAYMENTS

In order to receive payments on time you must learn and follow certain guidelines.

The most important aspect of filing insurance claims is to make sure that all of the information in the patient data and insurance fields are filled out properly. This is basically self-explanatory...always make sure that <u>every part of the claim form is properly filled out</u>. Even one number error will cause claim rejection. Other points to keep in mind:

1. **Fill out the section for radiographs when sending X-rays.** X-rays are always required for crowns, root canals, build-ups, periodontal treatments, surgical extractions, and for partial dentures. If no radiographs are being sent make sure that you mark <u>0</u> in this section.

2. **Double check that the patient is the patient and not the dependent or vice versa**

3. **Check the appropriate box for payment (or pre-authorization if this is the case)**

4. **Never make claims too extensive or complicated.** This means that you should separate your exam, X-ray, and cleaning claims from other claims that require X-rays and documentation. Category A procedures never require the consultant's review, whereas Category B and C will always be sent to the consultant (except for basic restorative procedures). If more than one root canal or periodontal procedure are performed in the same appointment try to bill these procedures on separate claim forms also...this will help expedite payment as they can be reviewed easier if the claim is smaller. To make this simple remember the following rule: bill composite restorations on one claim, bill root canals on another claim, bill perio. treatment on a separate claim, and bill your initial exam and X-rays on yet another claim (even if all of this work has been done in one appointment).

5. **Emergency exam claims must always have a narrative of the reason for the emergency and the procedures that were done. For example :**

    Patient presented with Right Facial Cellulitis secondary to abscessed tooth number 30. An incision and drainage procedure was performed and the patient was placed on antibiotics.

    Remember to bill the palliative treatment as well as the Limited XM and x-rays.

6. **Crown procedures that involve non-root canaled teeth must have pre-op X-ray along with explanation of why the crown was placed on the tooth:**

    the crown procedure for tooth #__ was done due to the extensive decay and cuspal fracture. The following cusps were fractured _____ and the extent of decay made it impossible to perform any other procedure but a full crown!

7. **Claims for partial dentures should have full arch P.A. x-rays (or panorex) as well as 5-year prognosis.** Dental charting of missing teeth should be completed.

8. Try to limit number of procedures to less than 5 per claim paper.

9. **Periodontal treatment should have charting, the minimum of bitewings, as well as a narrative of procedural steps followed during treatment. 5-year prognosis must be included.**

10. **Always keep track of the amount of insurance benefits that the patient has used up and know how much work can still be performed under insurance coverage.**

11. **THE MOST IMPORTANT PART OF CLAIMS PROCESSING AND RECEIVING PAYMENT IS TO FOLLOW UP RIGHT AWAY WHEN A CLAIM IS OVERDUE BY MORE THAN 30 DAYS. PATIENT MUST BE NOTIFIED AT THE 45 DAY INTERVAL.**

12. **Never accept the patient's attitude of "Oh, my insurance will pay!"** Patients must always be reminded of their responsibility regarding their claim. It is usually very helpful to get the patient involved in overdue claims, especially when they contact their employer regarding

the status of payment. The more the carrier is hassled the more likely that an overdue claim will get the attention that it deserves.

Different insurance companies have different contracts. What one covers, another may not. Sometimes it is a matter of trial and error when trying to figure out what is a covered benefit. Here's a few more helpful pointers to help you maximize benefits (READ SLOWLY):

1. Avoid four month recalls, except for patients that have had documented periodontal treatment in the past. Use code 04910 (perio cleaning) for patients with previous periodontal treatment who need to come in every four months. Advise the patient that they may be responsible for at least one cleaning, every third appointment. Also, a 4910 includes the fee for the exam.

2. Avoid taking bitewings every six months. Bitewings are normally covered only once a year. A full set of X-rays consists of at least 14 films, including bitewings. Panorex will not be covered along with a full set. A Panorex plus bitewings should equal the fee for a full set.

3. Fluoride can be given only once per year, for patients under 18.

4. Sealants are usually not covered. Under the age of 9, try code 1351.

5. Start your periodontal treatments, on new patients, with code 9110 (relief of pain - acute perio) or code 4355 (periodontal debridement), then go on to your perio codes.

6. Code periodontal treatments per quadrant by using code 4341 (scaling per quad) and noting the quadrant in the tooth column of the ADA form (i.e. UL, LL, UR, LR). Finish ALL quadrants of perio scaling within 90 days, or you may not get paid!!!

7. Periodontal treatments will normally need full mouth scaling (4341 x 4 quads). After 3 months of healing, if there is inadequate healing and resolution of inflammation, you must consider further treatment or refer out..

8. If the patient needs periosteal surgery following scaling, consider this a separate procedure and **wait at least 90 days before you sharpen your blades**. Code 4240 is used for flap surgery. You will get reduced payment for it if your perform it before 90 days following scaling and root planing. You may also want to finish your periodontal treatment program with an occlusal adjustment (code 9952). Just make sure that you are not delivering a crown or appliance at the same time or the insurance company will think that your adjustment is meant for the crown or appliance. And don't forget: you have to wait 90 days before you can do your first 4910.

9. Be careful of placing crowns on non-root-canaled teeth. You need photos and good X-rays to show pre-op condition. Document need (i.e. fractured cusps, loss of anatomy, gross caries, etc.). Fractured cusps!!!

10. Emergency exams are limited exams (140) when providing any services (extractions, drainage, etc.)

11. Porcelain inlays, onlays, veneers, and other esthetic advancements are hard to reimburse. Prior them, or better yet: do full crowns!

12. Posterior composites are often covered at the expense of amalgams. We charge patients the difference (in most cases this is usually at least 50% more than the amalgam fee; I add at least $50 to and above the normal co-pays per restoration). Keep this in mind when collecting co-payments. Insist on payment at time of service. Pay to play!!!

13. Code 9110 (relief of pain) can be used for many different visits. Obviously it cannot be used with a 7110 (extraction) or 2940 (sedative filling). Palliative treatment must be followed up with completion of therapy. Code 9110 should be used for emergency visits.

14. Denture/Partial repairs and relines can be done every three years. Do them!!!

15. Prosthodontic replacements are benefits once every 5 years. Crowns may be 10 years. Don't replace partials, or dentures unless you are sure that they are at least 5 years old. Always authorize these and crowns also. If there is malpractice involved, prior!!! Bridgework, partials, and dentures require documentation that gives dates of initial placement or reason for replacement. It should also include dates of extraction of teeth being replaced. Don't forget to send full mouth, mounted X-rays. If you plan on doing a bridge this year and a partial next year, in the same arch, you will only get paid for one or the other. Usually - the partial.

16. Current insurance websites allow you to do Pre-Determinations quickly.. As long as you have verified eligibility and waiting periods, bread and butter dentistry should be covered, without problems. But always authorize crowns, bridges, partials, dentures, bite splints, and periodontal treatments.

17. Bite Splints are covered only if they are done to prevent further destruction of the dentition (i.e. enamel fractures and attrition due to bruxism). Code 9940. Do not document joint or muscular problems...these are medical conditions! TMJ treatment is not covered by dental insurance, but you can get coverage through the medical carrier. Use an ADA form or HCFA 1500 and submit it to the medical carrier (use ADA code 9940 or ICD9 code 7880, along with a detailed narrative letter explaining your diagnosis and treatment). Bite splints are covered by dental insurance as long as there is damage to the dentition and/or there is periodontal fremitus.

18. Consider partials as alternative benefits when planning to do bridges. If the patient has missing molars #30 and #31 on the right side, and you want to replace #19 with a fixed bridge #18-20 on the left side, the carrier will only pay for a partial due to the edentulous condition on the right side.

19. Get reimbursed for photos: use code 471. Take photos of broken, non-root-canaled teeth, calculus deposits not evident on X-rays, and periodontal inflammation not diagnosable on X-rays. Take photos of any condition you may want to show the dental consultant in order to facilitate prompt payment.

20. Charges for prosthodontics and other multiple appointment procedures become liabilities on dates that they are started. Although liability begins at the first appointment, the carrier will pay for a denture or crown when it is actually delivered. Be careful in December and January. Some companies may use the start date as the date when services were performed, even though you may not finish the work until January. The carrier will not pay until the work is seated but will use the start date when considering benefits allowable. If you plan to use January's benefits (next year's benefits) don't start the bridge in December. Wait until January.

21. For patients with double coverage, coordinate benefits by realizing which insurance is primary. If one of the carriers has a non-duplication of benefit provision, then this insurance will not coordinate benefits as a secondary (it will only pay as the primary, and never as a secondary). Inform your patients to make their primary insurance the one which has this provision.

22. Crowns are covered only for reasons of breakdown and loss of anatomy. They are not covered to improve aesthetics, increase/decrease crown length, change occlusal plane, or place attachments.

23. Code 4341 is for SRP of 1 quad (5 or more teeth) while code 4342 covers up to 3 teeth of SRP.

24. Charges for X-rays are covered up to the fee of a full mouth series, no matter how many you decide to take. If you want to take a Panorex, do it on a separate visit. Panorex plus bitewings and PA.s equals a full set.

25. Bill for your study models (code 470).

26. Makes sure you document the type of alloy used for your PFM crowns. Have the lab supply you with the sticker of the alloy content used during fabrication, for each and every patient. Use appropriate codes. If your lab used a base alloy, you cannot charge using code 02790 (noble metal).

27. Bill for polpotomies (code 3220) when you relieve pain and refer the root canal. Do not bill if you are going to finish the root canal, however bill the 3220 if the patient does not return for the completion of the started endo. Remember: liability starts when you commence the procedure.

28. Get your patient involved in the process of obtaining benefits.

29. All ADA codes are treatment codes, not diagnostic codes like physicians use.

30. Always document the reason for the work: fracture, recurrent decay, open margins, infection, etc. Avoid restoring discolorations, abrasions, attrition, erosion, decalcifications, enamel defects, for insurance purposes. Insurance contracts are set up to cover subscribers for the basics of caries, fractures, periodontal infection, NOT natural aging processes or congenital anomalies.

31. If a patient cannot pay their co-pay write the following on the claim form: "Amount billed is our UCR fee...patient refuses to share in the cost of treatment." Never waive the patient co-pay. This is illegal and in some states, punishable by law.

32. If you are trying to bill for a workman's compensation claim, let the patient's lawyer get you the money. Get pre-authorization in writing and lay the goose egg on the patient's attorney.

33. Crown lengthening (code 4249) is not paid if performed at the same time with the crown. Do it as a separate procedure. Learn to do crown lengthening!!!

34. Try code 2960 for chairside laminate and 2962 for lab porcelain laminate.

Remember the following suggestions:

1. One root canal, core, and crown will exhaust over 75% of most contracts.
2. Pay attention to maximum coverage at all times.
3. Attempt to stretch out dental treatment over more than one year in order to not exhaust benefits.
4. Be available from October to November to complete dental treatment and maximize insurance benefits...when January rolls around you have two years worth of dental insurance to work with.
5. Watch out for Saturday appointments (verify insurance before the patient comes in for their appointment).
6. Never get into the frame of mind that "insurance will take care of it."
7. Learn how to verify eligibility.
8. Keep a list of all insurance companies and telephone numbers. Keep these log-ins as Favorites on your internet explorer bar.
9. Try to maintain a list of the customary fees that insurance companies pay for different employers...the same insurance carrier may have different fee reimbursement for different companies.
10. Educate your patients in regard to all of the fees, regardless of insurance coverage. Collection problems start with lack of patient communication and education.
11. Learn to properly document your outgoing claims. Always double-check your staff's work - deficiencies or errors will be your responsibility. If you sign on the bottom line, you become responsible!
12. Follow up on overdue claims (30 days past due) immediately...get the patient involved in the reimbursement problem. Get patients to call their employment benefit office or talk to the insurance company personally.

13. Collect all fees at time of service - don't get in the habit of "billing" patients.

Last, but not least, determine your fees according to your management style, your work schedule, the fees in your area, and your overhead. Although it is illegal for you to discuss fees with other colleagues, you can research fee reports published by The Bureau of Economic and Behavioral Research (available from the ADA) and investigate the prices charged by your colleagues. If every practitioner in your area is charging $100 for an extraction and you want to charge $200, you may have a problem. You must stay competitive. Make yourself available to larger segments of the population by not being known as an expensive dentist. Review chapter 9 (Finances) and figure out your hourly overhead. Then time yourself on all procedures and figure out what you should charge, per each procedure, in order to be profitable and stay ahead of your competition. Since recent graduates are at least half as slow as established practitioners, it may be hard to figure out a profitable fee schedule, based on hourly overhead. What takes me an hour to complete amounts to $200 of overhead, while a new graduate needs three hours ($600 of overhead). The difference is limited profit for the young dentist, but the fees should not be drastically different, when you take into account the competition and the usual and customary fees in your region.

Another eye opener that you should know about is the fact that insurance companies keep PROFILES on all doctors. They know what type of services you perform and how much you perform. They also know the quality of your work. Big brother is watching you, whether you know it or not. You will be audited if you exit the " norms."

If you need more help with your insurance and financial education please research the information on our website: www.dentalofficemanagementprogram.com

IF YOU HAVE FAILED TO PLAN THAN YOU HAVE PLANNED TO FAIL

CHAPTER 18
COLLECTING YOUR MONEY

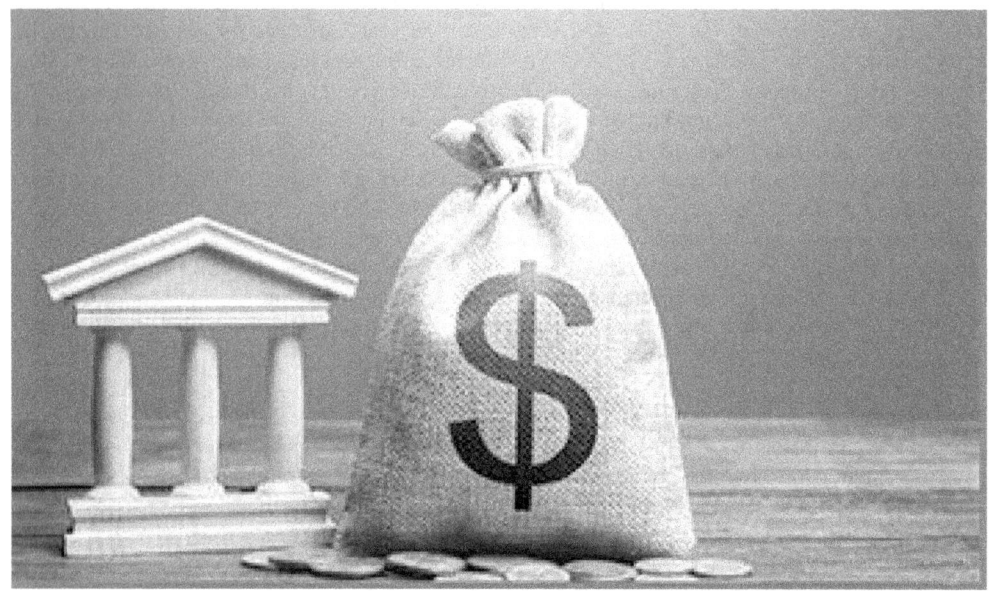

Now that you have learned to do everything the right way you need to get paid. You have improved your communication skills, you have gained patient trust/case acceptance, you have finalized your treatment plan, and you have discussed all insurance coverage and financial obligations. Once you complete the dental care, you have to realize that your next paycheck depends on whether or not you will get paid for all of the hard work that you have just completed. It is up to you and your staff to make sure that patients pay you for your efforts.

Even if you diligently follow all of the correct steps in patient education and clinical care you are going to run into difficulties when it comes to collecting your money. This will not be the rule, but the exception, if you have taken the time to communicate with your patients. Do not take a lazy approach to collections, whether you are an owner or associate. You must be involved in the process of getting paid!

This chapter is going to show you one of the most important aspects of maintaining a profitable career and an efficient practice. It has been copied from our management program.

Your Office Policy should be "Payment Due When Services are Rendered".

No other collection procedures are necessary if this is accomplished with each patient. Obviously this will not be the case every time. Some patients will give excuses as to why they cannot pay upon completion of procedure. The chances of this happening can be diminished if patients are aware of their balance and estimate of work to be completed, before the treatment is begun. Patients must always be made aware of what is expected of them before the procedure begins. Payment plans must be arranged accordingly and the doctor consulted each and every time that payments may become problematic. For those patients who are receiving simple treatments and payment plans are NOT allowed, you must make certain that they are able to pay their fee.

"Mr. Patient, I understand that you are receiving a (one surface filling on tooth 30 today). I wanted to let you know that the fee for the service is $___ and that it will be due upon completion."

What patients remember as they leave the office is usually what they remember most about you and your practice. This will affect how they will talk to others about you and your practice. The patient's exit can become an awkward situation when it comes time to discuss payment for the services rendered, especially if pre-treatment payment arrangements and treatment plans have not been completed and discussed with them. The only way you can avoid an unpleasant situation is to be knowledgeable and confident about your fees and your treatment plans. The staff may feel apologetic or reluctant about asking for payment if the importance of obtaining payment is not understood, and if finances have not been previously discussed.

Everyone in the office must understand the high cost of keeping the office running, irrespective of their employment status within that office. This involves knowing about expenses such as rent, insurance, equipment, lab fees, payroll, etc. The practice's fees are justified by all of these expenses. The electric company does not accept payment plans, neither does the telephone giant. Therefore, it is crucial to your existence to try and collect money at the time of treatment, while the services are still fresh in the patient's mind. Allowing time to lapse between services and collection results in decreased chances for payment.

Do not get into the habit of sending statements to your patients in order to collect what is owed to you. Statements should only be used for collecting unpaid insurance money and other payment problems. Your bill will usually get tossed in the garbage, so **you should never count on statements to collect your money.**

Once you have finalized your treatment plan and financial arrangements, the final step should be very simple.

There are several techniques employed in the process of dismissing the patient. You, the doctor, should not be involved in any of these procedures. However, I do recommend that you get familiar with fees and treatment plans, and not be afraid to discuss finances with patients - **BEFORE YOU PICK UP THE INSTRUMENTS**.

Do not follow the ignorant advice of so many consultants that stress a hands-off approach to the doctor discussing fees with patients. It is simple and logical for the doctor to be able to quote fees and prices to patients. Do not be afraid to tell patients how much your services cost! Feel comfortable doing it! Be proud of your fees! But do not be involved in the process of collecting money, at the completion of treatment, unless your staff is sick and you are the only one left in the office (in that case put on the hat of a banker and firmly ask for payment). Allow your front desk to do this and have them follow the suggestions listed in the appendix of this book.

You will actually spend most of your staff's efforts attempting to collect from those demons that we call insurance carriers. You must remember that insurance companies do not make their millions by paying out benefits...they make their money be floating premiums and delaying payments, while they earn interest on this money. Therefore, the longer that they take to pay you, the more money that they are actually making. Do not get frustrated with delays and rejections. Do everything possible to collect insurance money that your patients so rightfully deserve. Exhaust all of your efforts and educate yourself constantly about the changes in the insurance industry. Re-read the previous chapter.

Once you understand all of the different insurance contracts, clauses, exclusions, and ridicules you should not have a hard time collecting what you bill. If you do get rejections then it is usually because you either missed some form of documentation or there is a clause in the patient's contract that eliminates the service being billed. Helpful suggestions for...

Insurance Rejections:

1. Rebill appropriately.
2. Call patient immediately and have them pursue matter with employer and insurance.
3. Send more information, if required.
4. Send copy of signed form of Office Policy Regarding Insurance to patient to remind them of their responsibility for payment. Double check and make sure that all fees and treatment plans have been discussed, and all efforts towards rebilling have been made, before you irritate them.

Unpaid Claims

1. Anything unpaid over 30 days is becoming delinquent.
2. Contact patient by phone and have them call employer and insurance company.
3. Contact insurance company and inquire regarding the status of claim.
4. Resubmit claim, if necessary, with more information
5. At the 45 day interval, the account is delinquent....patient must be advised again of their responsibility and insurance company must be contacted (ask to speak to a consultant or manager) - address all rebills in the name of this person. Consider asking payment from patient!

How to Contact Patient (Delegate to Front Desk)

"Mrs. Patient, this is _____ calling from Dr. _____'s office. I wanted to advise you of the fact that the statement which I sent out to your insurance company for the treatment you had performed on the _____ of _____ has not been processed and we have not

received payment. We have allowed your insurance _____ days to process this claim yet we have not received anything back from them. I have to advise you at this time to contact your insurance and your employer regarding this claim because I will have to turn payment over to you personally, since this payment has become delinquent."

(advise patient of any resubmits you have made and any other pertinent information and send them the signed Office Policy Regarding Insurance Form).

WHEN ALL ELSE FAILS...

COLLECTING OVERDUE ACCOUNTS FROM PATIENTS

If all of your above efforts have failed you and you come to the point where the account has gone beyond normal time limits, you must get tough and business-like in your approach to getting paid. The most important aspect of collecting overdue accounts is TIMING. The longer you give a patient to pay, the less likely that you will receive payment. Collecting accounts by phone is usually the most effective way of getting the job done. Letters and statements are usually ignored, and are more expensive and time consuming.

Therefore, the faster your staff get on the phone about a delinquent account, the more likely it is that you will get paid. This means starting at 30 days, at 45 days, and turning over to collections at 90 days. Allow a designated staff member to do this, and do not get involved in the process, unless the patient wants to talk to you and/or they may be having problems with the dental work that you completed.

10% of your debtors are going to pay without problem after a phone call. The remainder will try to play games with you and purposely make your life miserable. Follow the next guideline to help collect money. Also keep in mind that about 10% of debtors may not be paying due to the fact that they may be unhappy with the services provided to them. If there exists a "real" dental problem that may be hampering the patient's dental health, and the patient feels that it may be due to the work completed on them, then it is important to get the patient back for an evaluation to determine what the problem is. If the patient refuses to come for an exam then consult with your malpractice carrier.

75% of the other debtors will stall payments but you will eventually get them to pay. The remainder of the debtors **(5%)** will never pay.

When talking to patients your staff must develop a sense of smartness so that they can distinguish between the people who have the funds but are unwilling to pay, and the patients who may actually be going through some tough times. Your aim is to find out the real reason why they have not paid. A salaried employee with full benefits should be able to make payments, while a part-time worker at a fast food restaurant will have difficulty. Research the account before the first phone call, including the treatment performed, their health history, and the treatment to be completed yet. Try not to waste your time on the "dead-beats". Be persistent on the people who can and will pay - the number will be a lot higher than you think. Follow the guidelines in the appendix of this book.

Remember that none of the above is necessary once you become familiar with insurance, treatment plans, patient education, and staff development. If you are in a practice where your collection problems amount to more than 2% of your gross income there is a problem with patient communication and policies. Patients will pay you once they understand what their responsibility is and what the value of their work is. Lack of patient education and information leads to collection problems.

If you do decide to turn your collection problems over to a collection agency, follow this advice: FORGET IT! You will waste your money and time. Hire an experienced collection attorney and let him/her handle your deadbeats. Realize that you will have to give up 30% of the money and you will receive a lot of negative word-of-mouth during this process. Consider chasing only large amounts (above $350) and writing off the smaller, non-collectible accounts. At Christmas time, have a charity event and grant amnesty to all of your small collection accounts. Invite these patients back into the practice, starting with a clean slate. Just make sure you get pre-payment next time around. You will attract more bees with honey!

If you need more help with your insurance and financial education please research the information on our website: www.dentalofficemanagementprogram.com

WATCH OUT FOR BIG PROBLEMS BECAUSE THEY HIDE OPPORTUNITIES

YOUR INCOME WILL EVENTUALLY REFLECT YOUR VALUE

YOUR BIGGEST ASSET IS YOUR REPUTATION

CHAPTER 19
BROKEN APPOINTMENTS, BROKEN HEARTS

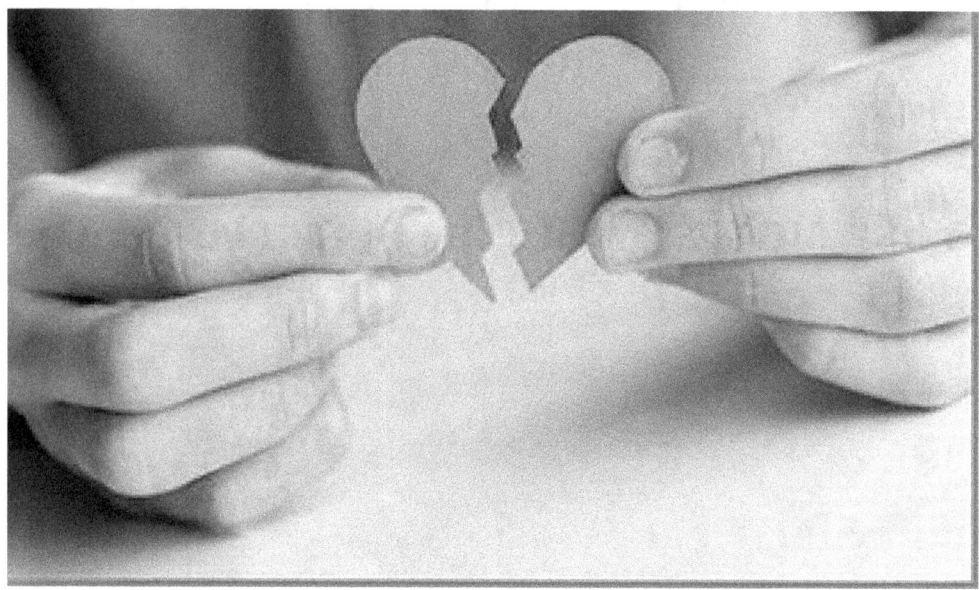

Appointment cancellations are one of the biggest headaches for most practitioners. Patients break appointments for numerous reasons. You must know some of these factors in order to be able to deal with this problem. Open appointment times will increase your overhead and cut into your profit margins. Again, this chapter is re-printed from our management system. Share this chapter with your employees. Study and apply these principles in your practice.

WHY DO PATIENTS BREAK THEIR APPOINTMENTS?

1. FEAR (BEING AFRAID OF THE DENTIST)

Any excuse that the patient can conceive before their appointment will give them a major reason to delay their treatment, and not show up for their appointment. A traffic jam, lack of parking, or a sore throat can quickly become a major obstacle and provide an "easy escape route."

Call the patient immediately and show concern.

"Mr./Mrs.___ you had an appointment with Dr. ____ at ____ o'clock today. We were worried that something may have happened to you."

2. PAYMENT PROBLEMS OR DIFFICULTIES

If patient responds that they had no money today to pay for their services, then respond:

"Oh, I'm terribly sorry to hear that. If you would like, I can sit down with you and discuss the different types of payment plans that we offer. This will make it easier for you to receive the care that you need."

(use good judgment when offering payment plans)

3. INCONVENIENT APPOINTMENT TIME

Change appointment time accordingly.

"I understand Mrs. Smith. Let me reschedule that appointment time for your right now so that you don't keep delaying that work that you need to have completed."

4. STAFF OR DOCTOR DISLIKE

Believe it or not, some people are not going to feel comfortable with you. It could be the way you look or talk - or it could be the result of deeper problems that which you need to address. The most common reasons include:

- **The needle hurt or the doctor was too rough.**
- **The work was not explained and was of poor quality.**
- **They were kept waiting.**
- **Appointments were not changed professionally.**
- **You ran behind schedule and ruined their day.**
- **They were not able to get appointments soon enough.**

Other reasons that patients may be leaving your office are:

- The staff did not talk to the patient, nobody listened to them, and staff was stuck-up.
- The doctor was impatient and did not explain things.
- The staff did not look professional, did not remember names, and everyone was cranky.

5. COMMUNICATION DEFICIENCIES AND POOR PHONE TACTICS

A script is what your staff says during critical patient contact and phone conversations. You should attempt to follow the same principles in order to help eliminate confusion, improper education and bad patient relations. The words that you use and they way you use them reflects professionalism and affects whether or not your staff will make that one or two extra appointments per day.

WORDS TO AVOID   INSTEAD SAY:

OPENING..............................*The doctor can see you at* _____

BOOKED..............................*Our appointments are usually reserved 3-4 weeks in advance*

SQUEEZE IN..........................*I can talk to the doctor about opening this time for you*

HAVE YOU BEEN HERE BEFORE..............................*When was the last time you saw the doctor?*

CHECK-UP..............................*Examination*

DRILL..............................*High speed preparation of tooth*

DEPOSIT..............................*Laboratory fees*

PAIN..............................*Discomfort*

WE'RE RUNNING LATE........*The doctor had a few unexpected patient emergencies and therefore the schedule is slightly interrupted*

6. NOT APPLYING SCRIPTS AND POLICIES

If you do not "teach" your patients about your policies then you are doomed to fail!!! Again, remember the communication process, the treatment plan, and the financial arrangements. If these have been completed, you have hurdled over your major obstacles.

EFFECTIVE WAYS TO REDUCE BROKEN AND NO-SHOW APPOINTMENTS

1. Try not to schedule the patient weeks in advance.
2. Remind patients of the importance of their dental needs.
3. Emphasize the value of reserved time.
4. Show respect for the patient's time (never keep patients waiting).
5. Advise patients of your office policies (charge frequent offenders, or invite them out of your practice...cancellations cost you money!).
6. Use the phrase **"We're looking forward to seeing you at __ on __ We have reserved a full hour of the doctor's time for you."**
7. Use Back-up List to fill in open times. This list should also include patients that would like to come in earlier than their appointed time.

8. Set limits on accepting excuses.
9. <u>When a patient calls</u> to cancel an appointment, reschedule the appointment right away.

"I really appreciate you calling Mr./Mrs.__, let me reschedule that appointment for you right now. I have the same time available on ____ the ___ ."

<u>When calling a patient</u> about a broken appointment and they do not wish to reschedule, your staff must ask questions to determine the problem. Most people who are dissatisfied with your office will give you the following excuse:

" I just don't have the time right now to come in."

You must respond by trying to find out if finances are a problem. If this is not the case, then respond:

"Is there anything that may have made you feel uncomfortable about our office?"

If YES,

"May I ask for your help as to the problem so that we don't make the same mistake again?"

if NO,

"I'm sorry you were not pleased...if there's anything I can do to help please let me know."

Do not reschedule frequent offenders with reserved appointments. Use Back-up, non-reserved times or consider charging a deposit fee to make their next appointment.

Follow the guideline on the following pages to deal with broken, canceled, and no-show appointments. Share these pearls with your staff.

THE KEYS TO REDUCING BROKEN APPOINTMENTS

SIMPLE STRATEGIES TOWARDS MAINTAINING A BUSY, SMOOTH FLOWING SCHEDULE

PUTTING THE PLAN INTO ACTION

Continue the patient education process when confirming their appointments.

confirm appointments: night before on weekdays; Sunday night for Mondays

how to confirm: clarify office policies, explain the "exclusivity" of the appointment

"Mr./Mrs.___, Good evening, this is ___calling from Dr. ___'s office! How are you?......That's great to hear. I just wanted to give you a friendly reminder about your appointment tomorrow at ___o'clock. The doctor wanted me to call and make sure that you will be able to keep this appointment, because we have scheduled a full hour of the doctor's time for you."

Patients think that you are like all the rest of the doctors. They believe that you will keep them waiting in your reception area for a while, and then you will see them for a short appointment. Stress to the patient that you have reserved one hour of uninterrupted time that the doctor will spend with them on their treatment. When they show up for their appointment seat them right away and make sure that you spend that "quality" time with them.

Follow these guidelines to deal with different situations, and reduce the number of broken appointments.

Patient cancels appointment:

response: express disappointment and worry about their dental problems!

if patient gives you a legitimate excuse:

"Gee, Mrs.____ I know that the doctor will be extremely disappointed with this change. The doctor was looking forward to seeing you tomorrow to get started on some of the work you need to have completed. Is there anything I can do to help you keep this appointment?"

if NO:

"Let me see when I can find another appointment for your treatment. I can reserve a time for you at __ on ___, but unfortunately this will be the only chance that I will be able to reserve an hour of the doctor's time for you."

If the patient does not give you a legitimate excuse (such as the "I don't have time right now" excuse) follow the previous guideline to find out if this patient was dissatisfied with our office. Of course do not reschedule if you feel that this patient does not want to return to your office.

Patient Cancels Frequently

"Mrs. __ I'm sorry to hear that, but this is your 2nd/3rd change in your appointment time. These changes are interfering with the treatment that the doctor had planned for you, and they are also a problem to our schedule. Our high demand from other patients means that I will need to make a special note and call you as soon as an appointment becomes available."

Place patient on the Back-Up list. Consider charging a minimum of half of your hourly overhead for patients that break appointments frequently. At my office we insist upon "deposits" before we schedule another such appointment. We will gladly schedule another appointment for a deposit of $100 per each hour reserved. If they show up the money goes towards their treatment. If they fail their appointment they forfeit the deposit. Accept credit cards to make it easier when doing this transaction over the telephone.

Chronically Late Patients

Schedule them 15 minutes earlier than the time you give them. Be understanding of unusual circumstances, but emphasize your policies.

"It's very important for you to be on time Mrs.__ because the doctor may not be able to complete the work you need and he/she will not cut corners to rush through your treatment. This will only mean more appointments for you, and we will be unable to keep rescheduling your appointments since this will interfere with other patient's appointments....the doctor's time is in great demand from many patients.."

DEALING WITH NO-SHOWS

Call within 5 minutes of being late. Don't wait longer because they may get the impression that we don't care whether they show up.

"Hi Mrs.___ this is ___calling from Dr. ___'s office. Is everything all right? We were worried about you because you did not show up for your ___o'clock appointment."

If patient states that they are on their way, respond:

"Let me put you on hold, Mrs.___ while I check with the doctor to see if we can still complete your treatment in the time that is left."

Check with the doctor and <u>if it is already too late</u> to start the work,

"I'm sorry Mrs.___ but the doctor does not feel that he can properly perform the treatment that you require in the amount of time that you have left for your appointment. I will be happy to reschedule your appointment at no charge this time. However, if you fail to make your next appointment, I will be unable to reschedule your time again."

Be understanding of unusual circumstances (i.e. snowstorm, car problems, traffic, babysitter,etc.)

PLACE EMPHASIS ON OFFICE POLICIES WHILE MAKING NEXT APPOINTMENT

Prime Time Appointments

Mr./Mrs.___ it's very important for you not to change the appointment that was scheduled for you. Changing your time will interfere with your needed treatment. The appointment time that I gave you is in great demand from all of our patients. I cannot guarantee that I can reschedule the same time for you if you miss this appointment. Availability of these time slots is very limited."

Long Appointments

"Mr./Mrs.___ we normally don't schedule such long appointments. However, the doctor feels that due to the complexity of your treatment he will need ample time to make sure that your work is properly completed. If you have to cancel your appointment with less than a 48 hour notice, I will be unable to reschedule such a lengthy appointment time for you."

At my office we do not schedule long appointments (over 2 hours) without a deposit. Since prosthodontic work involves co-payment, we require deposits before the work is begun. A minimum of $250 must be paid before the appointment is scheduled. If they fail their appointment the deposit is lost and must be re-paid. <u>You should also consider scheduling the</u>

longer appointment times either at the beginning of the day, or at the end of the day. This way, if the patient cancels, your day is not ruined.

As the doctor you should be aware of cancellation problems. You should always personally tell the patient how important it is to **RESERVE** your time in order to complete their work. Never tell patients that you only need a few minutes to do their work, even if you think you can complete the dentistry in a short time. Stress the importance of finding the time to do their work and the importance for them to keep their appointments.

Don't deal with idiots! Charge them for broken appointments and invite them out of your practice. Patients that break appointments, for no apparent reasons, do not deserve your time and care.

DON'T ALLOW OTHERS TO CHOOSE YOUR ATTITUDE

DO BUSINESS WITH YOUR PATIENTS WHENEVER POSSIBLE

IMPROVE ONE THING EACH DAY

CHOOSE TO LOVE YOUR PROFESSION AND YOU WILL NOT HAVE TO WORK A DAY IN YOUR LIFE

If you need more help with your patient communication, sales, and scheduling education please research the information on our website:
www.dentalofficemanagementprogram.com

CHAPTER 20
THE SPECIALTY ZONE

As you are developing your professional knowledge and expertise, attempt to develop a good working relationship with your local specialists. <u>Try to visit each specialty office at least once per month</u>. I used to spend two days per month with my endodontist friend. I also like to keep in close contact with my oral surgeon. I always try to stay on top of endodontic and oral surgery techniques. These are the most profitable procedures that you will perform. If your specialist is not open to allowing you to visit on a regular basis, then find another specialist that you can develop a better working relationship with. Try to learn clinical and communication skills from all of the specialists you come into contact with. Here is a quick list of the professionals that you must seek:

1. Oral surgeon
2. Endodontist
3. Orthodontist
4. Physical Therapist
5. Family Practitioner
6. Chiropractor
7. Prosthodontist
8. Pedodontist

Make sure that you take the time to evaluate your specialists:

1. Education and Continuing Education
2. Philosophy of Practice
3. Staff
4. Working hours (including emergency care)
5. Fees

In order to provide your patients with full service family dentistry you must not be afraid to perform the basic bread & butter dental procedures: composites, root canals, prosthetics, and oral surgery. Most practitioners are timid and afraid to venture into developing the necessary clinical skills required to provide some of these services. In particular, endodontics and oral surgery! If you are timid to provide these services because you're afraid that the lawyer down the street is waiting to skin your hide, then you may be sorry for wasting 8 years of education. Don't be afraid! Practice on extracted teeth, if you have to...but, just do it!

At the sake of being crass, I was having a conversation with one of my cardiologist friends about medicine and modern care. After a long talk he started to laugh and said to me: "You're talking about teeth right?" and I looked at him and I said: "You are right, it's just a tooth, nobody will die from losing a tooth!"

While we are taught to cherish and worship teeth the majority of human beings do NOT place as much importance on their dentition as you do. Losing a tooth is not life and death to most people. So, be comfortable with the fact that you may lose or mess up a few teeth along the way and you should accept that fact of life, especially since you are "practicing." That is why they call your office a dental "practice".

Here's a real reason why you have to consider Endo and OS: a molar root canal, core, and crown (procedures that can be easily accomplished in less than 2 hours) can add $500,000 to your yearly income. And all you need to do is only one per day. Add a daily set of wisdom teeth to the equation and you are close to $1million dollars a year. Not bad for about 15 hours of clinical work per week! Don't be afraid to be successful! Diagnose it and sell it! Then, just do it!

HIGHER PRICES DO NOT MEAN HIGHER QUALITY

IF IT SOUNDS TOO GOOD TO BE TRUE, IT IS

IF SOMEONE WANTS TO TEACH YOU HOW TO MAKE MONEY THEIR WAY, YOU WILL BE MAKING THEM MONEY

CHAPTER 21
OVERCOMING FEAR

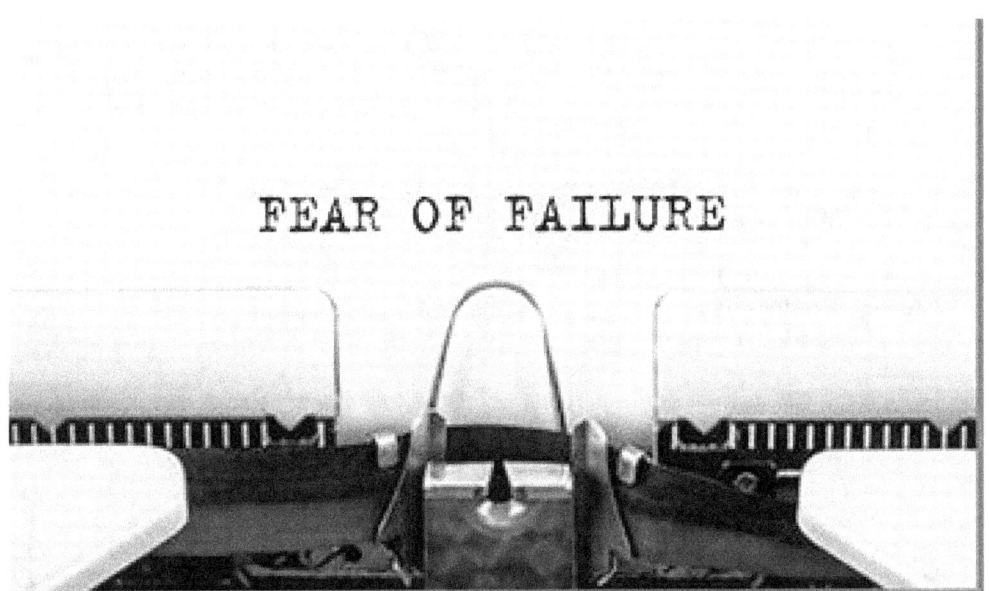

I wanted to devote an entire chapter to this subject because it is one of the most important areas of practice and patient management that all practitioners have to master. **It is the cornerstone of a successful practitioner and a profitable practice**. Almost all of your patients will have some inherent degree of fear of the dentist. Some patients are so afraid that they will do everything possible to avoid your office. It is your responsibility to overcome your patients' fears and apprehensions. When I first started out in practice over 90% of my patients were delaying treatment because of fear. After five years of building my reputation I have found that my patients have come to trust my care so much that fear is no longer a big obstacle in my practice. I now deal more with financial and scheduling difficulties than I do with fear. Once you learn to develop your skills of being a gentle dentist, your reputation will quickly travel through the community. It will be your best advertising!!!

I handle all of my fearful patients with a few basic strategies. Drugs, drugs, and more drugs!!! Just kidding! Although I regularly dispense Valium, I have come to learn that most patients simply want to know how you are going to deal with their problem of being afraid. I always take the time to explain to my patients how topical anesthetic works and emphasize how we take the time to make sure that they are fully anesthetized before I begin any work. Of course, I always suggest Valium and nitrous to all of these patients to help them overcome the jitters. Usually after a few nitrous sessions, most of these patients come to find out that there is nothing to fear. Most fearful patients turn out to be my best and most courageous patients. There is nothing wrong with dispensing 15 mg of Valium one hour before appointment time for your fearful souls. You should also offer at least 60% nitrous during their visit. You will have one cooperative puppy on your hands.

I always re-stress to the patient how we anesthetize their teeth and make sure that the nerves are "dead" before we begin the work. Most patients don't want to hear the word needle, so I always explain to them that *"we place a little anesthetic right next to the tooth."* Don't use the word "needle!" There are times when I am working on upper teeth that I will bet the patient the cost of their visit if they feel anything. I have lost only one bet in 30 years, to a palatal canal during a root canal procedure on #14.

The other part of my fearful coaching clinic depends on adequate patient education. **Most of your patients' fears stem from:**

1. **A previous bad dental experience.**
2. **Thinking that they are not going to be in control of their situation.**
3. **Not knowing what to expect.**

The main aspect of helping your patients overcome their dental fear is your ability to empathize with them and let them know that you understand how they feel.

"Mr. Patient, I have had numerous dental procedures in my own mouth and I know how you feel because I am also very afraid to have dental work done. However, this fear is usually only a result of our inability to be in control and being afraid of the unknown. We will not do anything at our office to surprise you and we will always explain to you what we are doing. You will always be in control and you will always know what our next step will be."

Do not say "There is nothing to fear." The last dentist probably said the same thing.

Once you have crossed the bridge and the patient is ready to proceed with treatment, you must back-up your sales pitch and deliver quality, gentle dentistry. Get in the habit of using a lot of topical anesthetic. Dry the tissue with cotton and let the darn thing sit on the vestibule, or palate, for at least two minutes before you inject. When you are ready to inject remember this word: SLOW!!! Go easy, little buckaroo, because if you are in a hurry to inject you will cause pain. For upper procedures, I always pull the upper cheek taught, as I inject, and wiggle the vestibule as I deliver the local. I never penetrate more than 2 mm. and it usually takes at least 90 seconds to deliver one carpule. If I am doing full quadrant restorations I will slowly place the anesthetics in one spot and "ladder" my next injection points slowly across, using previously injected tissue to work my way over. Once I have delivered one carpule per 2 or 3 teeth, I wait 2 minutes and then I slowly deliver another carpule, deeper into the vestibule in order to let the anesthetic reach the apex of the teeth. Therefore, 2 carpules per 2 or 3 teeth is ample to numb this number. Make sure that the second injection goes high into the vestibule.

If I am doing perio surgery, root canals, or wisdom extractions, I always numb the palate. This can cause discomfort. To eliminate pain, you must allow at least 2 minutes for the topical to work. Before you inject, place the end of your mirror handle on the site and apply pressure. This will cause pressure anesthesia. Inject slowly, penetrating only 1 or 2 mm., at first. After 20 to 30 sec. penetrate another 1 or 2 mm. and then take a 2 minute break before you inject close to the bone. Usually 1/3 of carpule is enough to numb 1/3 of the palate (2 maxillary nerves and one incisive nerve make up the entire palate). Don't be in a rush!!!

For lower injections, I advise the patient that they may feel a little mosquito bite. I do not lie and tell them that it is going to be totally painless. Lowers always sting just a little bit, even if you do everything else correctly. The more you wiggle the jaw and/or head the more you can distract the patient. Again, go slow!!! Begin to deposit anesthetic as soon as you penetrate the first 2 mm of tissue. Stop, pull the needle back and massage the area for 20 seconds. Then go slow as you penetrate deeper. Make sure that you never hit the bone! Deliver one carpule, wait 2 minutes, and give another carpule. Then, wait 3 minutes, and check for the signs. Ask your patient what feels number, lip or tongue!? Of course, if they say tongue, you must deliver anesthetic a little higher and more posteriorly in the triangle. If the patient still does not feel entirely numb, try again. Always do a buccal nerve block along with the IANV block and normally I also do PDL injections when starting root canals.

Sometimes it is a good idea to inject high and close to the last molar, without going too far back. I call this my wisdom tooth injection. The buccal nerve can be anesthetized in this area and you may just be lucky to catch the other branches as well. I have had many cases where the patient did not get numb after 2 Regulars and 3 Gow-Gates applications, only to get numb after a high and shallow injection. The 30 gauge needle barely penetrates 1/2 of the way, but I make sure that I am coming from the opposite side of the mouth upon delivery.

Try to observe the direction of your needle. You should be angling from the opposite lip commisure into the pterygomandibular triangle region. Do not attempt to direct the syringe from the same side. To be able to get to the canal opening you need the right angle, otherwise your needle will bend and you will numb the parotid instead of the nerves. You will experience a few episodes of eyelid anesthesia with associated ear and parotid numbness. This is an indication of improper anesthetic placement. You have gone too far posteriorly!!

On the other hand, if the patient's lip is numb and the tongue is not, proceed to inject lower and maybe a little more posteriorly. This is especially true on young adults. After you have done a thousand lower blocks, you will begin to get a natural feel of the canal opening area. It is almost as though you have gone through the tissue with some resistance and suddenly you feel a little looseness at the tip of the needle. Sometimes you may encounter some resistance due to tight ligaments. You may actually feel like you have hit the bone when in fact you're stuck in a ligament. Don't be afraid to slowly keep penetrating! Just make sure that you maintain the same straight angle. Tight ligaments are always experienced on TMJ patients!

I use a 30 gauge needle for my first IANV and Buccal Block. Then I switch to a 27 gauge.. Try not to bend the needle after you have penetrated the tissue and do not change direction abruptly. Sure you may have to alter this rule once in a while but make sure that you don't end up with a broken needle inside your patient's tissues.

My first carpule of anesthetic with the 30 gauge is always Plain Citanest. This anesthetic has a neutral ph, therefore it does not sting upon contact with tissue, as do most of the other available anesthetics. Your patients will appreciate it! After the initial carpule has numbed the area, I inject Marcaine or Lidocaine to prolong the anesthesia. The Citanest is only used as a first injection.

There are times that you may find that no matter what you do the patient will not get numb. This usually happens in the following circumstances:

1. **When you have a female patient menstruating.** The hormonal changes in some women somehow change the body's tolerance to anesthetics during this period. This person will simply not numb. Politely and professionally ask your female patient if they are menstruating. If so, you may want to re-appoint in two weeks. This scenario happens infrequently, but I have come to learn that it is real, especially with my female patients undergoing estrogen therapy and/or experiencing hormonal imbalances. Watch out for menopause!

2. **When you have a patient that has a recent injury, to <u>any part of their body</u>.** Injury causes the body to release bradykinin, potassium, and arachidonic acid, which starts the depolarization of the adjacent nerves. This depolarization not only travels down the nerve but also affects other nerves, causing them to be sensitized. The blood vessels swell, while the sympathetic system revs itself up to high gear. Plasma leaks out of blood vessels and mast cells spread throughout the body. The consequential histamine release, and the white blood cell response to the injury, will render your anesthetic useless. If I notice any recent injury to my patient, I hold my breath for the results of the lower block. Sometimes I have to reschedule. This is also true for patients experiencing a bout with the flu or cold bug. The sympathetic discharge is sometimes too much to overcome!

3. **When you have patients that use recreational drugs**, or when they are taking narcotics or other pain medications for more than the last seven days. The nerve endings are so tolerated that the anesthetic will not block the sodium channels. The synapses are also so tolerated that the neurotransmitter is in constant activity. Never use Epinephrine with patients that have told you they use cocaine. If they don't numb with plain anesthetic then refer them to someone that does IV sedation dentistry!

4. **When your patient is so nervous and hyperactive** that your anesthetic is about as good as water. You must calm your patient down. A lot of your emergency patients may be in this state. That lower molar may be so painful and hyperemic that there is just no way you can numb it. Calm the patient, then worry about numbing the tooth. If you have to, prescribe medications, and re-appoint. Don't hurt the patient, unless they request that you proceed.

5. When the two-pack-a-day patient just finished half-a-pack before his appointment. **Smokers** have nerve endings that are so tolerated your Marcaine is practically useless. These patients have nerves that are firing even in their sleep. Today's anesthetic is just not strong enough to block the sodium channels.

6. When you have a **hay fever** patient and it is hay fever season. Good luck! The histamine release in the body will laugh at your Xylocaine. Wait until after the molds and funguses are frosted, or call their allergist.

7. Modern day **stressed-out Socialites**. Again, sympathetic overdrive. Calm the patient, calm the tooth!

8. Gallon **coffee drinkers**. About as difficult as smokers! Sympathetic toga party!

9. TMJ/Headache Patients. Remember that your headache/migraine patients are subclinical TMJ patients and they will cause a majority of your clinical problems. Learn to diagnose them. Stop their clenching first! Learn more about this subject as it will make your professional life a lot easier and really help you grow your practice if you learn even some simple basics on how to treat and stop clenching.

No matter what the situation, besides the above recommendations I have found a few things that can help you achieve success with anesthesia. Check with your state requirements for anesthesia and seriously consider taking some courses on this subject before you start doing these 2 protocols:

<u>1. Basic Sedation:</u> 15 mg. Valium one hour pre-op; 60% NO2 during appointment

<u>2. Moderate Sedation:</u> Keep these drugs in your office and have patient come 90 minutes before their appointment. They can wait in the reception area or you can block off their chair during the 90 minute sedation time. Take their BP and review their medical history closely. Then, Dispense the following cocktail:

Benadryl 50 mg
Atarax 25 mg
Triazolam .25 mg
After 90 minutes check their status and see if they are ready to proceed.

If the patient does not feel "relaxed" you can also administer 50% NO2 at this time but carefully monitor them with a finger Pulse Oximeter and take their BP every 15 minutes. You can get them into very deep sleep once you add NO2!

If you plan on doing Moderate Sedation you should have Log book with your medications and fill them out for each visit. Sedation Scheduling Check list

Name of Patient_____ Date_____
BP/P_____ Medical History_____ Instuctions Given_____
Your Signature_____

Make sure that all patients receive Written Instructions on what to do before their visit:

Patient _____. At your next visit you will be receving Sedation. Please be advised that you must not eat or drink any solids or fluids a minimum of 3 hours before your visit. You must have someone pick you up from the office approximately ___ hrs after your arrival. You may drive yourself to the appointment but you cannot drive after. Please let us know if you have ever had an adverse reaction to: Benadryl, Atarax, or Triazolam

3. IV Sedation: get licensed and hire a nurse anesthetist if you want to do this.

CHAPTER 22
PEDODONTICS

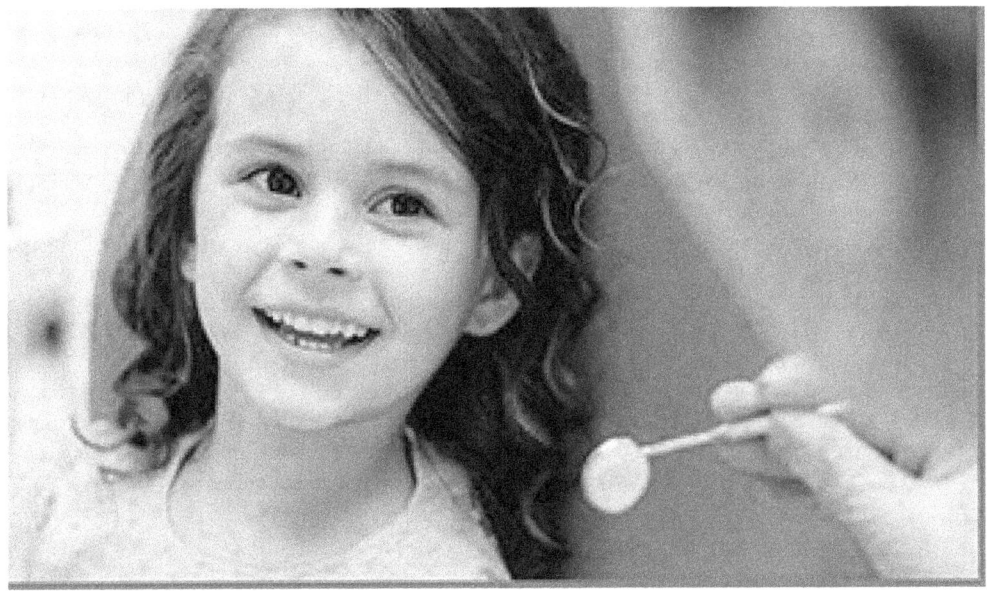

The ability to deal with children successfully is often a challenging aspect of being a dentist. Many practices have found that their growth has resulted directly as a result of good pediatric skills. Many mothers will send their children to you in order to test the waters. Meet the needs of the children and you will have the entire family coming to your office.

If you don't like children don't attempt to treat them, other than providing cleanings and exams. If you decide to treat children then you must be able to control your temper and stay in charge of your senses. You must learn how to deal with different child behavior before you can offer pedodontic services. Managing children depends on your ability to prevent behavior problems and turn negative experiences into future confidence.

In order to develop pediatric skills you should spend some time with your specialist. Learn about the different personalities/behaviors of children:

The shy child wants to be given diverted attention. Let them know that it is perfectly O.K. to be afraid while talking to the parent. Don't pay direct attention to this child. Give them infrequent attention and let them come out of their shell.

The uncontrollable child should not be confronted. Let them scream, kick, and howl. Refer!

The <u>defiant child</u> should not be confronted. Let them hit the chair and refuse to cooperate. Allow them to display negative behavior and encourage them to do so until they get tired of it. If they don't cooperate after 15 minutes, REFER!!!

Never scold, threaten, or humiliate children. Accept their behavior! If you decide to treat, follow a few of these suggestions:

1. Use Ativan 1 mg. one hour preoperatively.
2. Use NO2.
3. Work fast.
4. Extract all necrotic teeth (don't do polpotomies on necrotic pulps).
5. Don't fix primary teeth after 8 years of age, or earlier, if development is advanced. Why fix small decay that will not penetrate the pulp before the patient will lose the tooth?
6. Core material and composite are less traumatic, and just as good as a stainless steel crown, for broken down primaries. Composite polpotomies are also becoming more popular than eugenol polpotomies (remove the pulp chamber, etch, prime/bond, and seal with composite or core material). I have not done these so I cannot comment.
7. Pay attention to development and space problems.
8. Learn to not overtreat!
9. When you have to refer, explain to the parents that it is in the best interest of the child to seek the services of a pediatric specialist that is better equipped to handle their special needs. Never make it appear as though you do not want to take on the challenge.

HUG A BABY

TAKE A KID TO THE ZOO

KISS A SKINNED KNEE

IMMERSE YOURSELF IN YOUR CHILDREN'S LIVES

LISTEN TO CHILDREN

CHAPTER 23
EMERGENCY CARE

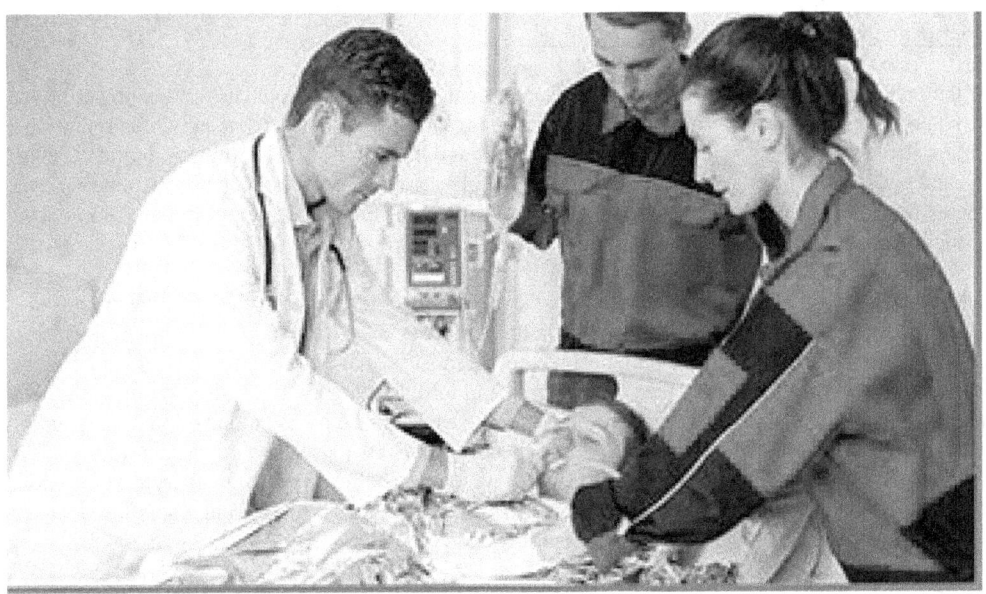

Emergency care is going to be your greatest practice builder. Appoint patients immediately and take care of their pain without delay. At my office, true emergency patients are seen pronto, Tonto! It takes five minutes to prepare their paperwork and confirm insurance, and it usually does not take longer than 10 minutes to alleviate their problem. Obviously there are those patients who do not qualify as real emergencies and we know how to handle these patients. Some patients simply want to be seen right away because it is convenient for them, and they will try to come up with some sort of ludicrous emergency need. Your front desk personnel should know how to handle these patients. Nevertheless, 90% of the patients who have an emergency should be seen immediately. The *cry-wolf* patients are also appointed promptly, but at our convenience. True emergencies (accidents, cellulitis, pain, fractures, and even broken dentures) are appointed immediately and we will break from a busy schedule to see them.

Training your assistants to handle the emergency patient is essential to being able to expedite care and stay on time. When a patient tells the assistant that they have pain on the upper right side, she should take a bitewing and P.A. of the area, without need for your directions. The bitewing is your most essential diagnostic aid because it helps you see clearly around crown margins and showd you depth of any decay present. Pas may show apical problems but they cannot indicate where the problem originates. The assistant should also prepare the room for necessary treatment. This is usually either an endo or surgery set-up. When you enter the operatory to see the patient, the assistant should have a differential diagnosis completed. This is not hard to do and does not require a DDS or DMD degree. After you meet the patient, complete the examination, numb the patient, return to what you were doing, and then come back and perform the palliative. Pulp extirpation should not take longer than 10 minutes, an extraction requires no more than 7 minutes, and even the most difficult surgical extraction can be done in under 30 minutes. If you want to refer, call the specialist and get them to see that patient right away (as in the time it takes for them to drive over to that office). <u>If your specialist will not see your patients right away, find a different one!</u>

If the patient does not wish to proceed with treatment, or visit the specialist, write a prescription. If you do not have the 10 minutes to treat, write a prescription, as long as the patient is not in dire straits. Do everything possible to assist that patient and take care of their problem, without delay. An exception to this rule may be the patient who has a "hot" tooth and is not responding to a lower block (review chapter 21). This patient will appreciate a later appointment, along with some medication (ATBs, Motrin, Benadryl, etc.).

At my office I see many emergencies who come from other offices where no treatment was rendered for their problem. Most of the time the patient is even told that there is nothing wrong. The problem is usually not the patient, but the diagnosis. I have done hundreds of root canals, cores, and crowns for patients who were in pain and told that there was nothing wrong with them by other practitioners. Take the time to diagnose the cause of the pain! Patients do not call and/or come to your office to interfere with your schedule. The last place anybody wants to visit is a dental office. When someone tells you that they have pain, believe them! Do everything possible to find the cause of the problem and get the patient comfortable. If the patient wants to come see you, they have a need. You should do everything possible to help them.

Denture patients are considered pseudo-emergencies, but we always fix their broken teeth, or bases, without delay. Most denture teeth can be fixed or replaced in less than 15 minutes. Broken denture bases require only about five minutes. A cold cure intraoral hard reline only requires 10 minutes. Broken clasps, or other extensive repairs, only require a 5 minute impression.

Here is some helpful advice for your emergency appointments. Use these suggestions to help make definitive diagnoses:

1. When a patient presents with pain and they cannot tell you where it's coming from, **think TMJ and Sinuses before you try to make any other confirmations**. TMJ and sinus problems can manifest as tooth aches. Review the XRs (especially the BWs and rule out pulpitis and fractured teeth. If you don't find anything obvious ask the patient AGAIN: do you suffer with headaches? Do you clench your teeth? Have you been in any accidents? These open your door towards possible TMJ diagnosis. Palpate the musculature and joints. If there are no apparent dental problems and you do NOT offer NTI therapy then instruct the patient to buy a soft mouthguard at the store and return for a splint. Our normal protocol is to deliver an NTI and prescribe Flexeril 10 mg h.s. If you don't know how to make an NTI, visit www.chairsidesplint.com and watch the videos on how to make these. It will change how you practice. In many cases, we deliver an NTI and won't even find the need for full coverage splints.

Sinuses can also cause upper, and sometimes lower teeth to ache. Patients that have allergies and sinus problems can present with non-specific dental pain especially in the upper molar area. Check the breathing clearance through the nostrils and palpate the maxillary sinuses for tenderness. Prescribe Tetracycline and OTC Afrin, if the sinuses are inflamed.

2. When a patient points to one tooth and tells you that it is the cause of their pain, they are usually right about 90% of the time. Check for decay and/or old restorations. Ask the patient about the symptoms: pain upon biting, sensitivity to cold/hot, constant aching, etc. **Constant throbbing indicates a necrotic pulp**. This tooth may or may not respond to cold and heat. If it does it will usually have lingering pain to either, or possibly be relieved by cold. A root canal is required, obviously! If the pain is only elicited by cold, ask how long it lasts. **Lingering pain (more than 20 seconds) indicates a pulp that is irreversibly inflamed and necrosing.** Root canal! Pain to cold that lasts for just a few seconds may indicate a pulpitis, but it can be reversed. Have them purchase some ACT Fluoride and Crest Sensitive Toothpaste or Sensodyne. If the tooth exhibits no deep decay, but has a large restoration, think of necrotic pulp (even if the amalgam is 20 years old). Many old amalgams have damaged pulps that have survived many years without symptoms. This is also true if there is any periodontal infection. Periodontal pathogens can travel through accessory canals and infect the pulp.

If the tooth is virgin and there is no periodontal problem, consider a vertical fracture (once you have ruled out TMJ and sinus problems). Take a Q-Tip, or Tooth Sleuth, and have the patient bite on each cusp <u>independently</u>. If the patient jumps when biting on any one of the cusps, suspect a possible vertical fracture on that cusp. Try to luxate that cusp and see if you can get it to move freely, in order to remove it. If not, relieve the occlusion and check in a few days. Some vertical fractures may not reveal themselves for a while, but they usually produce pain. Do not let your patients suffer - Extract, if the fracture is into the root system!

If none of the above is working out for you, consider a neighboring tooth or an offending tooth on the opposite arch, same side. Take more bitewings and search further. If you cannot find anything, refer back to suggestion #1 and start all over. It is almost impossible not to be able to diagnose the cause of dental pain. BWs are helpful especially when a patient thinks the problem is #14 but BW shows large decay on #18.

3. Take a few empty carpules of anesthetic. Fill them with water, put a QTip in them and freeze them. Use these ice sticks as your #1 diagnostic tool, especially when you are trying to decide whether a tooth is still healthy. Get in the habit of doing this during your regular examinations, especially before you begin crowns on non-root-canaled teeth. **Don't crown necrotic teeth!** Use these ice sticks during all visits to help you check the pulp status. The air/water syringe is also useful, but not as precise.

The entire diagnostic process should not take longer than 2 minutes and 35 seconds, unless you may be dealing with a rare neuro/muscular problem. 99.9% of your emergencies will fall under one of the above suggestions. Don't complicate things.

INSTALL FIRE AND CARBON MONOXIDE DETECTORS

KEEP SPARE KEYS

BUY JUMPER CABLES

BUY A TOOL-BOX FOR YOUR TRUNK

BUY A FIRE EXTINGUISHER

LEARN HOW TO USE A FIRE EXTINGUISHER

CHAPTER 24
CLINICAL BASICS

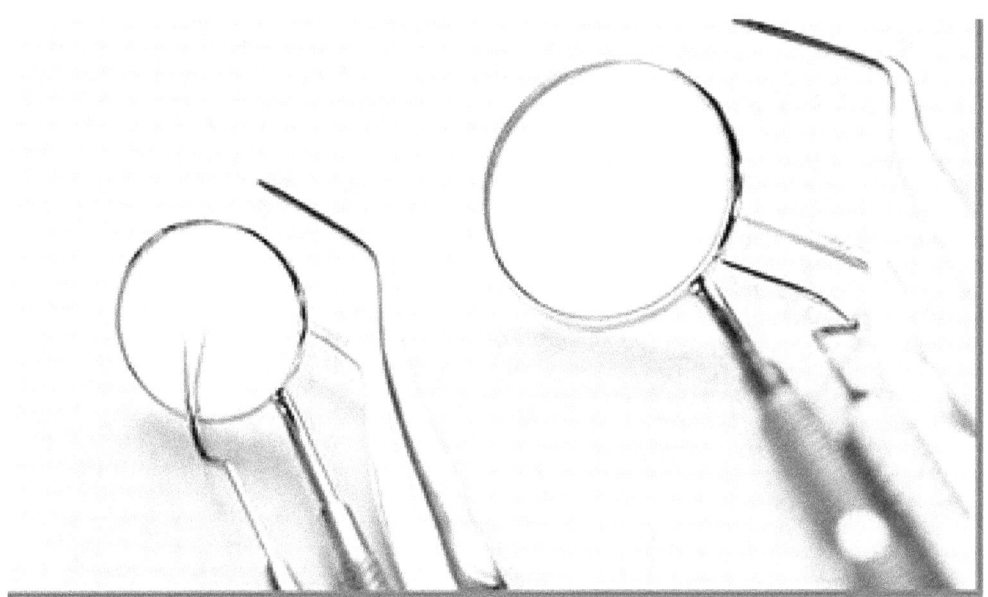

No matter what procedure you are going to perform for a patient there is one step you must always take before you begin: **check the periodontal condition and the occlusion**. This is a critical step for all restorative procedures. The success of your clinical work depends on healthy gum tissues and stable occlusion. Don't begin any crown preps or veneers, especially on anterior teeth, without addressing the periodontal status and occlusal harmony. Future gingival recession and exposed crown margins will affect your work. Occlusal instability will lead to breakdowns and failures. Take the time to plan your work! Remodel the house, only if the foundation is sound and the roof is not leaking.

Your clinical success depends on longevity and fit. The periodontal probe must be one of your main diagnostic tools. The articulating paper, along with correctly mounted study models, will be one of your blueprints. Follow this basic law of treatment planning before you take the gun out of the holster.

Plan to not fail!

WINNERS DO WHAT LOSERS DON'T

LEARN TO FIX DENTAL EQUIPMENT

DON'T BELIEVE PEOPLE THAT USE THE WORD 'HONEST' TOO MUCH

LEARN TO SAY NO

ACCEPT DISAPPOINTMENTS

PRACTICE EMPATHY

PROMISE BIG; DELIVER BIGGER

CHAPTER 25
THE RUBBER DAM

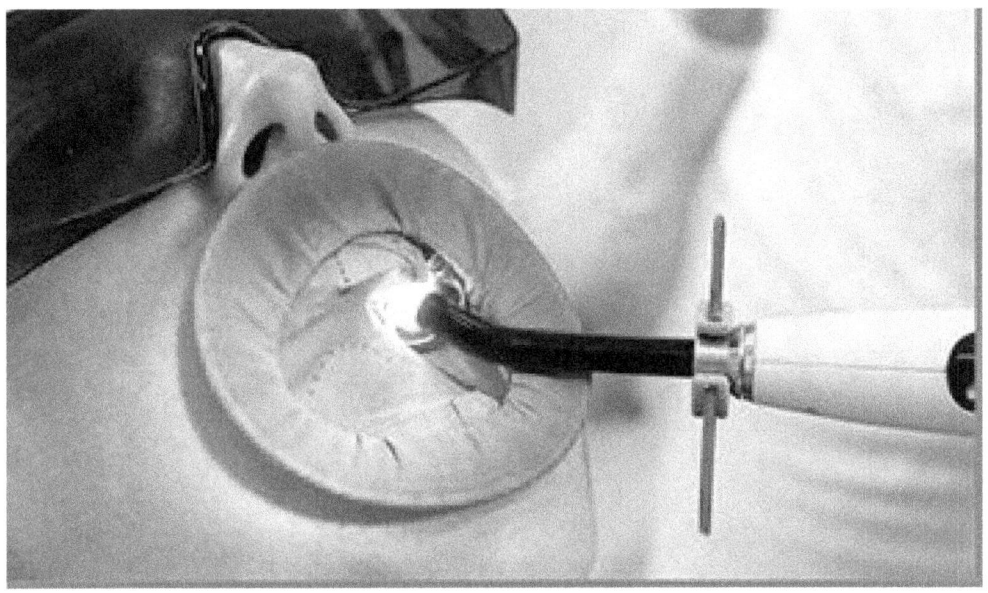

I read so many articles by well known experts who advocate the use of the rubber dam for virtually all clinical procedures. It is obvious that these guys are spending more time writing than they are performing dentistry. I love the rubber dam. The damn thing is the greatest invention since sliced bread, however I cannot always use it. This is especially true if I am working distal to a first molar and the patient has a tight vestibule, or small mouth. When I can use it, I do not hesitate to place it. The rubber dam saves me time and improves my vision and is great for root canals.

For the past few years we have been strictly using the DryShield. Best investment you will ever make!

If patient cannot tolerate the DryShield I will consider just using the rubber dam clamps with cotton rolls.

If you prefer rubber dams keep this in mind: the rubber part of the rubber dam is always the culprit of a few swear words. Make sure you purchase the thickest dam material available. If it tears or rips don't fight it...leave the clamp on and go! When I am able to place the dam without difficulty (especially true for anterior or premolar region work) I **try to ligate it to the opposite arch as much as possible**. In other words, if I am working on #20, I punch holes for the dam to go all the way across, to at least #27. If I am working on teeth #s 6 through 11, I will place the

163

dam from #4 through #13. You don't always have to punch individual holes. One large hole can serve to isolate three or more teeth. The more of the rubber dam that I can get on the teeth, the more clearance I have, and the easier it is to use. This gives me more working room and provides stability. It is also helpful to use some Vaseline to ease it over the teeth. Review your dental school books on this subject. You received more than ample information on this topic.

NEVER TELL ANYONE THEY LOOK TIRED

COMMIT TO CONSTANT SELF-IMPROVEMENT

RELAX

BE POSITIVE AND ENTHUSIASTIC

TAKE NO ACTION WHEN ANGRY

AVOID NEGATIVE PEOPLE

PRAY FOR WISDOM, NOT THINGS

CHAPTER 26
CARIES REMOVAL

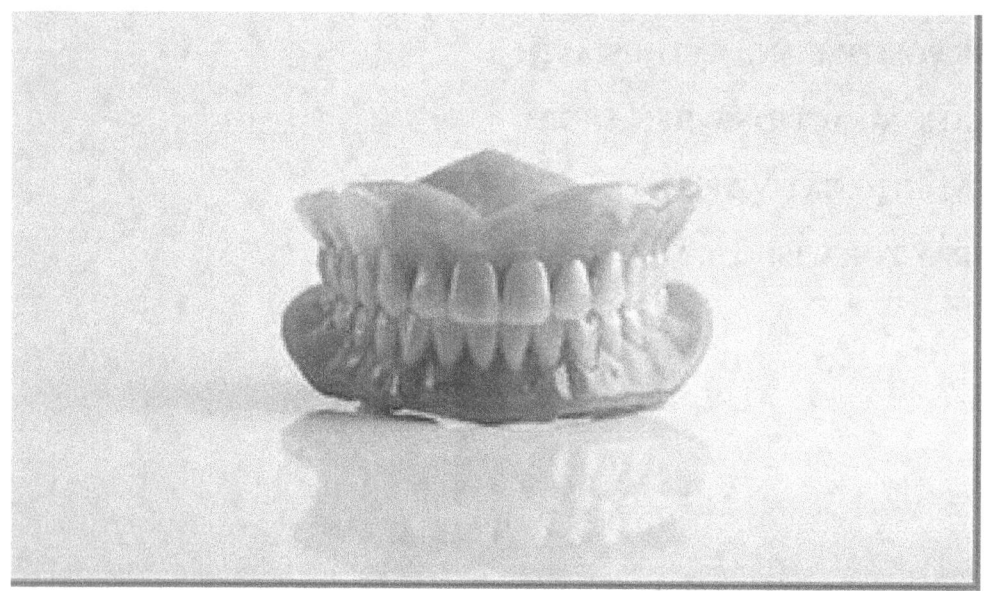

A few years ago I bet one of my associates that I would find decay on every one of his final preparations. I would be a rich man had he taken me up on the wager. So many practitioners gather around conference tables wondering about what materials they should be using for restorative work. The drawbacks do not begin with the restorative materials. **Clinical failures result, first and foremost, from inadequate caries removal.** Obviously, the other reasons are poor technique and lack of knowledge of the proper use of the dental materials.

One of the most important reasons that I can give you to get you to master the art of removing decay is the fact that incomplete caries removal leads to post-op sensitivity and unretentive fillings. Remove all of the decay, and if deep - root canal! Do not be afraid to get down and dirty and remove ALL of the decay. Indirect pulp caps do not work. CaOH is a tooth's worst enemy! Residual microbes (left from incomplete removal) leads to sensitivity, pulpitis, and necrosis. Strep Mutans could probably live under the Titanic, so don't believe that covering them with restorative material will suffocate them or destroy them. They're going to have a picnic under your amalgam or composite. Remember, those little buggers shit acid.

Caries removal is an art. It is the cornerstone of a successful dental practice. It is the main reason that you received a dental degree. Most of your dental school clinical curriculum was centered around caries removal and tooth preparation. This key element must not be forgotten in your private practice. Unfortunately, too many practitioners fail to realize its importance and do not serve their patients ethically and adequately. Effective and complete caries removal is not being practiced by a large number of practitioners.

The use of decay-detecting solutions is an integral part of mastering the art of caries removal. Purchase the individual caries detector microbrushes and use them for every restorative procedure Use it and you will be amazed at how much decay you are leaving behind in your preparations. This is especially true on crown preps!!!

The appropriate sequence and use of slow-speed round burs is important when cleaning out the tooth. Think of the caries as a funnel. You start at the wide end with a #6 bur and you must proceed to the tip of this funnel with progressively smaller burs (down to a #2). You cannot use one large bur to remove all of the decay. The #6 round bur cannot burrow down into the tip of the funnel. It will remove the large part of the decay, but the deeper caries will be left unblemished, because the larger burs will be rotating unto healthy enamel without penetrating down into the remaining caries. **You must progressively use smaller round burs to get to the bottom of the caries.** When you think that you have finished caries removal, take an even smaller round bur and go back over the decay. You may just be surprised to find more decay, deeper down. Just be careful when you get to a #2 because you can actually remove healthy dentin and expose the pulp. Light stroke with lots of irrigation!

The use of antimicrobial agents to disinfect and kill the bacteria residing in the cavity has been in wide use. More on this topic in the next chapter.

Never forget to use your round burs to remove decay on your crown margins. You may think that the margins are clean but more often than not you will leave decay on the margins!

The longevity and comfort of your dental work depends on complete caries removal. If you follow the above steps and complete your caries removal completely, the remainder of your restorative work will be easier, smoother, and long-lasting. Take time to remove the decay!!!

Besides the caries detectors, you should also use magnification. Work with loupes. They will improve your work, save your eyes, and take stress out of your neck and back.

CHAPTER 27
POST-OP SENSITIVITY

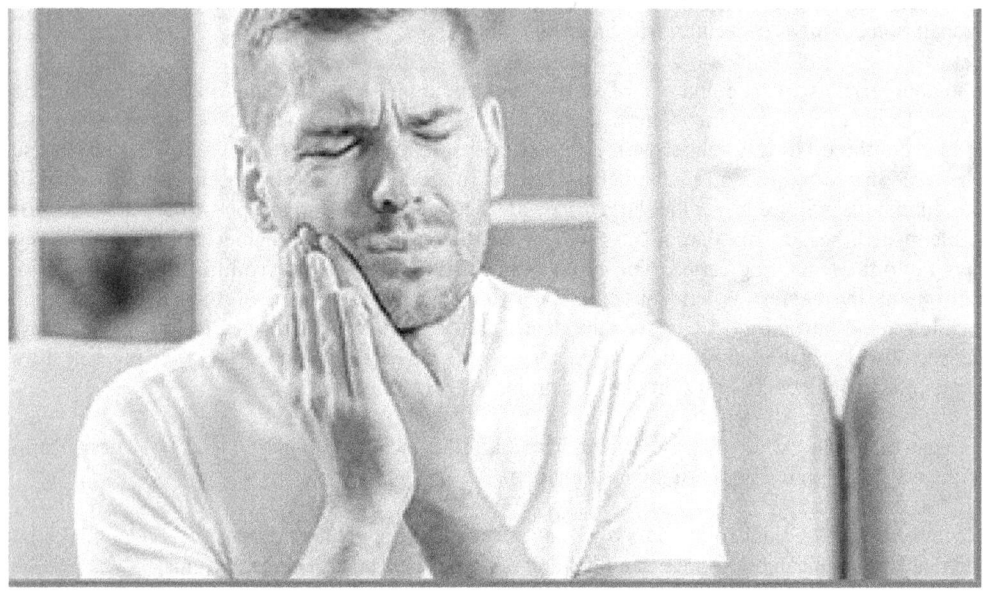

You must take into consideration what the patient will experience and feel after you are done with the work. Post-op sensitivity is the biggest problem that you will encounter in your practice. This discomfort can normally last up to four weeks. This a negative comment for you and your staff. Many practitioners begin to doubt their skills, and their materials, when this happens. Although you cannot completely eliminate all post-op sensitivity, you must take the appropriate steps to diminish the length of time and duration of this problem.

The reason that teeth get sensitive is due to an inflammation of the pulp. An inflamed pulp has high chances of necrosing because it has poor healing properties, due to its minimal blood flow.

Pulpitis can happen for a number of reasons. Here are the basic reasons and some simple solutions:

1. **Inadequate caries removal**. Always remove the caries completely. Make caries removal an important and integral part of all of your clinical work. It is also helpful to evaluate your radiographs for caries extent. Bitewings are very educative in terms of blue-printing your way into cavity depth preparation. Never rely upon appearance when evaluating your caries removal. When in doubt, take a smaller round-bur through the jungle, one more time. Just when you think that you are done, take an even smaller round bur and buzz through the

dentin some more. You will be surprised at how many times you will still get decay out. USE CARIES DETECTOR! USE IT EVERY TIME!!!

2. **Being afraid of deep cavities.** A lot of young dentists are afraid of deep cavities. I have even seen some practitioners attempt to put three sedative fillings on teeth that should have received a root canal ten years ago. Here's a golden rule that you should osmose into your cerebellum: if in doubt, root canal!!! Don't try any David Blaine routines. If your bitewings show a cavity in close proximity to the pulp, do the root canal. If you don't, you may just regret it later (especially if you have placed a $1000 crown on the tooth). A lot of deep carious teeth will still exhibit normal EPTs pre-operatively. However, many times after mechanical preparation, the chance of that tooth remaining healthy is slim. One of my basic criteria for not performing root canals on deep cavities is as follows: at least 1 mm. of sound dentin must remain, the EPT was normal, and I have carefully checked the caries removal. <u>I usually take a bitewing during preparation to determine exactly how much dentin I have left.</u>

3. **Burning the tooth.** Use copious amounts of water with your high-speed and cool your low-speed caries bur with water irrigation. Those darn low speeds don't seem like they can build up heat, but they sure do. <u>Keep the tooth cool!!!</u>

4. **Improper disinfection.** Mix some chlorhexidine (Peridex) with Bleach (5:1). Use this mixture to disinfect your teeth - we'll call it PB from here on. You can use Ultradent's LureLock brush tip/syringes for doing this. Clean and irrigate the tooth during and after preparation. Soaking the tooth with this mixture, during low speed caries removal, is a good way of scrubbing down the dentin. This mixture acts as an antibiotic which kills the bacteria harboring inside of the cavity. <u>You should also use this mixture during crown preparations and prior to crown cementation, as a cleanser.</u>

5. **Use Hemaseal or Gluma, followed by Ionoseal or Limelight when close to pulp.**

6. **Overheating the tooth.** Copious water should be coming out of your high speed during preparation. Also: your assistant should always be spraying the tooth with air/water when you are using round burs in the slow speed to remove decay. Never cut dentin without water irrigation!!!

7. **Overetching.** Be careful when you etch. Never etch for longer than 15-20 seconds when using 35% Phosphoric. You will melt the dentin and cause pulpitis.

8. **Dessicating the tooth.** Watch that air-water syringe. Don't desiccate!

9. **Failing to remove solvents.** Evaporate the acetone, or alcohol, from the primer/bond. After the second layer of primer/bond has been placed, **lightly** dry from a distance of about 6 inches away for around 3 seconds or less.

10. **Contamination.** Keep Moisture and saliva away! Watch your isolation!

11. **Inadequate condensation.** Take time to adequately fill the restorative material. Always use good condensation and avoid any possible voids. When placing composites pack slowly and

carefully to avoid air voids. Some experts agree that you have to place composites incrementally in order to avoid shrinkage and gap formation and therefore - sensitivity. I have not found this to be true. **You can bulk fill, believe it or not**. It will actually give you a better restoration, with less chances of air bubbles getting incorporated. More on this later.

12. **Undercuring of the primer/bond/bond.** Cure your primer/bond/bond carefully. Cure your composite slowly. More on this later.

13. Do not **overheat** when polishing composites. Use copious water and light strokes.

14. **High occlusion. Check the occlusion.** Bring patients back for re-adjustment, if necessary. Watch out for *stray cats* when doing composites. This material likes to flow and sometimes you can't see it sitting on functioning cusps or straying away from your preparation.

15. **Leaky temporaries**. Seal your temporaries. Use Luxatemp or Integrity with Temp-Bond NE and don't forget to use Hemaseal after finishing the prep.

16. **Dirty tooth**. Disinfect your crown preps with PB before cementing. Scrub them down and then seal the dentinal tubules one more time with Hemaseal just as though you were placing a composite restoration. Clean the tooth and seal the tubules, doc!

If you stop and think about what you are doing when you're working on a tooth you should have an easy time eliminating sensitivity. Keep the tooth cool and seal the dentinal tubules. Destroy the bacteria and compact your restorative material. Check your occlusion and don't desiccate the tooth. It's really not brain surgery!

A few words of wisdom about sealing the dentinal tubules. Dentinal tubules are about six times larger in size than bacteria. Have live bacteria...will travel, and irritate! Destroy the bacteria with your disinfectant and you have practically eliminated the bacterial problem from your equation. After you have bombarded the decay, you should etch the dentin and enamel for no more than 15 seconds. This removes the smear layer and part of the calcium matrix and gives you clean, ready-to-go dentin and enamel. The other effect of the etch on the dentin is that it collapses the tubules and the collagen which were held together by the calcium matrices. The tubules and the collagen need water in order to prevent collapse and closure. I use Optibond because I like the one-time use compules (prevents material from being degraded by air and frequent use/opening of the bottle) and also because it contains a water base so I don't need to worry about hydration. I don't use onding agents that have acetone and alcohol based solvents because of the need for water to re-hydrate the dentin. The H2O molecule also acts as a " taxi" for the bond. It shuttles the bond down into the dentinal tubules for optimal seal and bond strength. I also like using Hemaseal and Gluma as "desensitizers" because they allready have water as a solvent and therefore do not require a wet surface. There you have it. A full day course in one paragraph.

If you decide to use an acetone or alcohol based bonding agent then, wetting the dentin does not mean that you should fill the tooth with water before priming. All it takes is just a little wetness. After you rinse off the etch, place the high volume suction over the tooth, count to three, and you should have a wet tooth that is not full of water. If you want, you can dry the tooth and surrounding structures after rinsing the etch, dip your sponge-tip applicator brush in water, apply it to the dentin and enamel, and then use the primer/bond. Don't forget to place enough primer/bond to completely seal the tooth. This may take 2-3 layers. After you have applied the primer/bond WAIT 60 seconds to allow the primer/bond to get down into the tubules. Follow this with a **light** stream of air to evaporate the acetone, before curing. Hold the air/water syringe at least 5 inches away. Again, the high volume evacuator can also be used for this step. You know that you have completed the right technique when the dentin looks glossy, after curing it. If it does not look glossy you need more primer/bond. I normally apply a second light coat of Optibond before placing my composite.

The enamel also needs water before priming/bonding. I know that this sounds crazy for a lot of you who have been taught to keep the enamel dry. Your bond strength is improved if you slightly wet the enamel, before bonding it.

After complete curing, the dentin and enamel must be dry. I dry the tooth and all surrounding areas thoroughly, after the second cure, and before placing the composite.

It is very important to cure the primer/bond/bond thoroughly in order to prevent any pull-back or zipping. First, check the output of your curing light. Most manufacturer's recommendations for curing times are based on 500 mwa of light output.. For every 100 point decrease in light output you must double your curing time.

As long as you have a powerful light, the rest is easy. Think of your prime/bond as a magnet that holds together two train cars trying to go in opposite directions. First it must bond itself to the east-bound train (the dentin/enamel) and then to the west-bound train (the restorative material). If you fail to cure it completely you will not have adequate strength to keep the cars from separating. You must bombard the prime/bond with adequate curing light in order to make sure that it will have adequate strength to hold the cars together. This is usually at least 20 sec. with a new curing light.

Once the dentin and enamel have been sealed and bonded properly, the restorative material should have an easy time gluing itself into the bonded layer, and therefore the tooth. The next chapter will detail the restorative phase.

The Golden Rule: The better the bond, the less post-op sensitivity.

Another key aspect is to remember that your air/water syringe must not mix any water with air. Sometimes, when the O-ring gets old inside the syringe you will get water mixing in with your air. It is important to check this closely. Blow some air on a Kleenex. If it gets wet you have a problem because water contamination, after curing the prime/bond, will ruin your composite. The only time you need a little water is right before applying primer/bond to the dentin and enamel. At no other time should your tooth be wet, after the dentinal tubules have been sealed.

If you follow and think about the above recommendations your patients will be more comfortable and your phone will be ringing less. Your patients' comfort will reward you with better word-of-mouth and increased referrals. And remember - do not be afraid to do the root canal, when you have to!

CHAPTER 28
RESTORATIVE DENTAL WORK

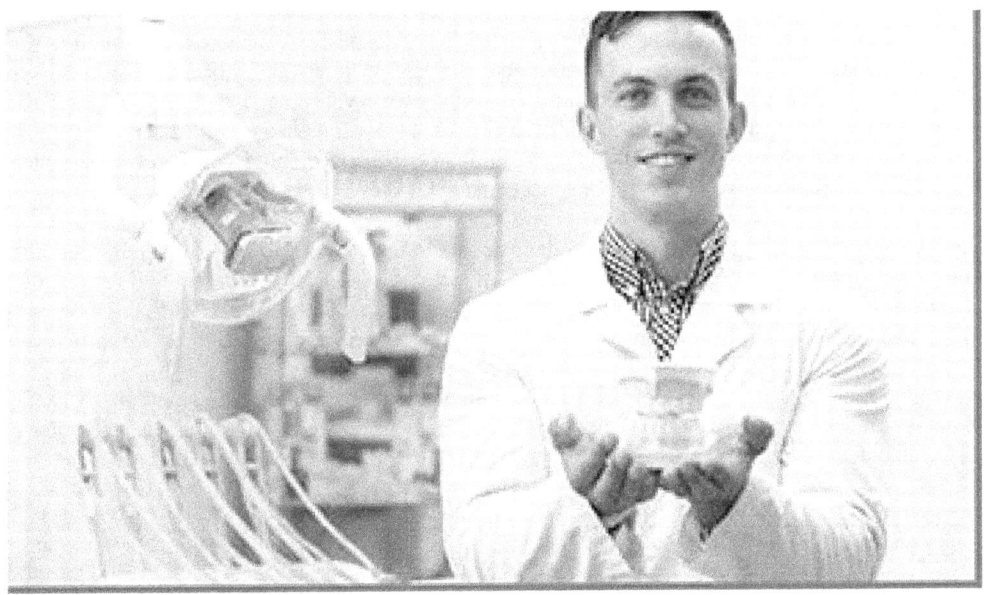

Quality restorations increase your self-esteem and strengthen your trust with patients. It promotes practice growth and professional success. Poorly fitted restorations lead to stress, professional set-backs, and bad patient relations. Patients know and can feel the quality of your work, whether you may think so or not.

Concentrate on simplifying your routine and avoiding unnecessary steps. However, you should not try to cut too many corners as you drill, fill, and bill. Rely upon your dental school basics and strive to improve your speed and coordination. Don't rush into cutting preps and filling them as fast as you can in a vain attempt to be profitable. Quality, Quickness, and simplification of your procedural steps come with experience and repetition. Here are a few extra helpful pointers:

1. Use your knowledge of cavity prep design to make your amalgams retentive <u>if you still choose to place amalgams</u>. Flare and reverse taper are your most important allies. Create a smooth pulpal floor and check your isthmus for adequate width and proper depth. Most amalgams fail due to isthmus fracture (secondary to shallow or narrow preparations). They also fail due to inadequate condensation. Once your preparation is adequately completed, take the time to condense the amalgam. Don't throw you amalgam carrier away!!! This is the best instrument that you have to help you place the amalgam in deep areas, such as cervicals. Don't be in a rush to get the amalgam in the tooth and pack it. Use incremental additions to slowly condense the amalgam and get a proper fill. **Learn to use your ball and anatomical**

burnishers as condensers...they help pack the amalgam against the sides of the preparation a lot better than most condensers. Sometimes I don't even use the condensers.

2. Don't forget to check your matrix placement, and use wedges tightly. Pay careful attention to the *mesials of upper premolars and molars*. The mesial concavity will make it hard to fit the band. Use your wedge to secure the band tightly, and take a post-op BW of these fillings to check your fill. Don't wait six months to check the adequacy of your work. Do it before the patient leaves, while they're still numb!!! Don't forget to run your explorer along cervicals and use it as a carver when necessary. Always check your facial and lingual areas for completeness of fill. Evaluate your interproximals for adequate contact. Patients will complain if they get food impaction from an open contact. Re-doing your work will reduce your income. Filling your restorations inadequately also causes sensitivity.

The basics of placing composites relies upon adequate isolation, knowledge of the materials, and sealing of the dentinal tubules. Water and saliva contamination will wreck your composites. Use rubber dams as much as possible, or carefully isolate with my previous recommendations. Improper dentinal sealing will cause post-op sensitivity and *gap formation*.

A single tooth composite restoration is a simple procedure. Pay careful attention to shade selection and caries removal. Since composites require no design form, it is easier to leave undetected decay behind.

To perform excellent composite restorations you must understand the mechanical properties of the composites. Curerntly I use only Omnichroma!

When you are bonding the composite into the primer/bond layer, which is bonded into the dentin/enamel, you have to consider what happens as you cure. If you bombard the composite with a strong curing light at the beginning of curing it is the same as dipping it in liquid nitrogen. It will crack, shrink and pull away from the primer/bond layer. Therefore, to compensate: wait at least 60 seconds after placing the bonding agent and then use your light slowly. Start from a few inches away and slowly get close to the material.

The moral of the story is that you can actually overcure your composite. You must cure your composite **slowly** in order to keep some elasticity into the material. The easiest way to do this is to cure for 20 seconds from about 4 inches away, at first. Allow the free radical reaction to begin, and wait about a minute before doing any more curing. You do not want to alter the modulus of elasticity of the material. If you cure it quickly you make the material brittle and it will shrink, crack, and pull away from the sealed dentinal layer. Again, stay a few inches away and don't hurry the process at the beginning.

How you fill the cavity preparation is also very important.

Incremental composite placement is NOT the way to fill....for small to medium sized restorations.

The sequence that I use for my posterior esthetic work depends on the size of the preparation. For small to medium preps you can obviously bond and fill in less than 30 sec.

When I pack large cavities I use Ionoseal over pulp horns and one incremental layer of composite which covers the pulpal floor and most of the dentinal surface area. This first layer coats the entire dentin. In interproximal areas (with matrix on) I will place a cervical layer of composite and cure this before adding more. Then I bulk fill the rest.

As a general rule, after the initial layer of composite has set, the tooth can be filled with composite in one **bulk delivery**. Don't be afraid to do so. You should overfill the margins and the tooth as a whole, but not excessively. This helps minimize shrinkage and voids at the margins. Of course you can still use incremental additions, if you want, just be careful about incorporating air voids because it is difficult not to do so. That is why bulk delivery is better. If I knew I could prevent voids with incremental additions I would probably still use this method, but I am realistic enough to realize that this is not always possible.

Some practitioners use two curing lights to speed up the curing process. This is a good method, but it should be used only after the initial free radical reaction has been set in motion by the first low exposure curing. Remember: you want to cure slowly, at first, to prevent the liquid nitrogen effect. After a few minutes, the free radicals have begun the hardening process and you can hit the composite with stronger light. However, you should never cure to the point where the light heats the tooth. As a general rule, I do not cure any composite for more than 30 seconds, and this is after I have waited five minutes from the initial low curing step. If you try to hurry a composite you will get sensitivity because you will have gap formation, which leads to fluid movement within the dentinal tubules.

The curing light does not completely harden or set the composite. It only starts a free radical reaction that actually takes about 24 hours to complete itself. Your composites will not reach a hard stage until the day after.

When you are ready to perform posterior composites, keep in mind all of the previous basics we talked about: healthy gums, tight wedging, complete caries removal, occlusion, etc. Using posterior composites has a benefit that amalgams do not offer. Your preparation can lack all defined criteria of design. As long as the caries is removed and you have access to fill, you're ready to go. For the most part, composite preparations are much more conservative in nature than amalgam preparations. You still need flare, in order to trim and evaluate the margins in the future, however the other criteria can be forgotten.

The one problem you may encounter with posterior composites is a lack of a good, tight contact. To eliminate this problem use the Palodent or Garrison system. Wedge the tooth as tightly as possible, use the thinnest metal matrix band available, and burnish the band into the proximal of the adjacent tooth. I like to use metal bands because they hold up better than the clear ones and they can be burnished into the adjacent tooth. Another helpful suggestion is to pack the composite (whatever material you choose) into the cervical about half-way up the tooth. If your preparation is small then place the composite and **hold the ball burnisher against the band**, pushing into the adjacent tooth. Cure the composite, while holding the ball burnisher. Make sure you do not imbed the burnisher into the composite. The hardened composite now holds the band snugly against the adjacent tooth half-way up from the cervical and you can finish filling the remaining half.

When performing multiple anterior composites, attempt to finish one restoration at a time. Normally, when I am restoring over four teeth in the anterior region I will finish all preps and caries removal. After this I will seal/bond, restore, and trim **one tooth at a time**. This may seem more time consuming, however it pays off since you don't have to spend a lot of time polishing and trimming at the end. Your restorations will also look better, since it is easier to trim interproximals one tooth at a time, instead of trying to trim them after they are all filled. The embrasures and contact areas will also be easier to restore.

It is also helpful to pack some cord around the cervicals of teeth when doing multiple composites. This helps prevent bleeding, especially if a rubber dam is not being used. Bleeding may happen even in a healthy mouth. You must do everything possible to prevent contamination. **Never use metal containing hemostatic agents/astringents such as Astringedent** - they will discolor the gingiva, stain your composites, and make your post-op results look unprofessional. The astringent will not wash off, even when you are waiting on your lab a few weeks. **Use clear astringent.**

Composites are easy to trim with football shaped 12-fluted burs and fine diamonds. I personally like the fine diamonds! Always double check the occlusion. Just when you think that you have finished trimming and polishing your posterior composites, go back and do it again. It is hard to see the white composites sticking to areas of the tooth that you had no intention of filling in the first place. Extra composite on a functioning cusp could cause severe pulpal irritation, secondary to high occlusion, after the patient leaves the office. **Always check subgingivally...bonding agents love to run and hide in the sulcus areas. It may appear as though you have a nice smooth margin finish, when in fact you may just be running your explorer over excess composite or bonding agent.** In the anterior you can use a gingival retractor to pull back the gum and allow you to visualize what is happening down there. Leaving overhangs will cause periodontal defects. Your lawyer will love you!

I always insist on a second polishing appointment for all of my composite restorations, if the patient feels any bite discrepancies or sensitivity. I insist that my patients return three days after the appointment to complete any necessary adjustment.

For final composite finishing I use plastic saucer shaped and flame shaped polishing cups along with Polishing Paste. Before dismissing the patient, double and triple check the occlusion. I also blow the tooth dry and carefully check for any composite "strays" on cusps or other areas.

As far as marginal seal and leakage is concerned, think about your technique and caries removal. Composites last a long time in mouths that have good hygiene as long as they were placed properly and carefully. Don't expect your composites to outlast amalgam, despite the bonding characteristics. If you get 12 years out of them, be happy.

As far as onlays and inlays are concerned: I have not offered them in a long time. 3 Surface restorations are usually composites, 4 surface composites depend on occlusion, and anything above 4 surfaces usually warrants a crown.

Concentrate your efforts on procedures that you can do easily, often, and with more patient acceptance.

DON'T ALLOW OTHERS TO CHOOSE YOUR ATTITUDE

DO BUSINESS WITH YOUR PATIENTS WHENEVER POSSIBLE

IMPROVE ONE THING EACH DAY

CHOOSE TO LOVE YOUR PROFESSION AND YOU WILL NOT HAVE TO WORK A DAY IN YOUR LIFE

CHAPTER 29
ROOT CANALS

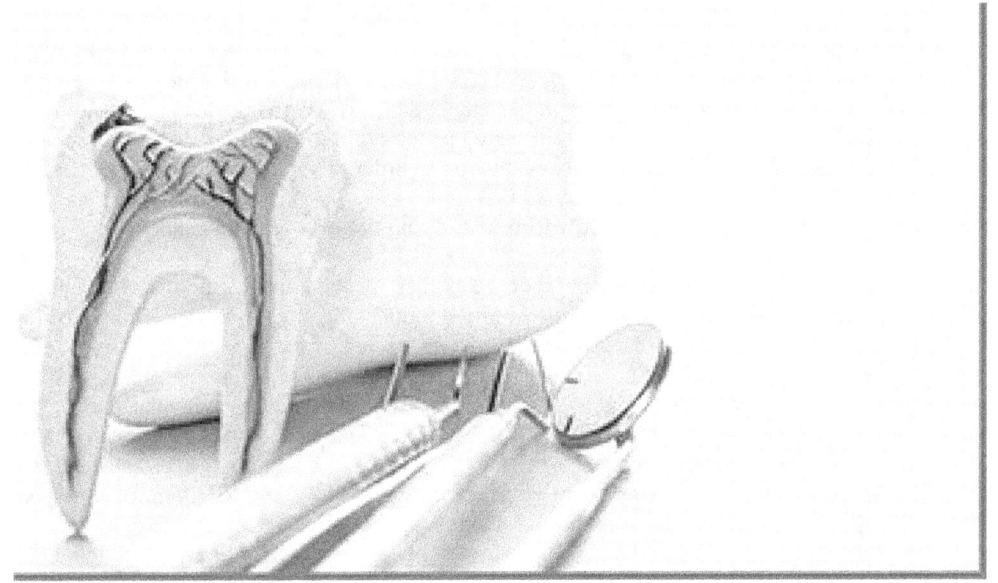

You know that deep cavity that you thought you were going to put an MOD amalgam on? The one you're probably going to encounter within the next few days of clinical work? Prepare to get your files out.

Too many practitioners are afraid to diagnose the need for root canals. Don't be fearful when presenting the possibility of root canal therapy to your patients. It will save you from embarrassment and win your patient's trust. If you don't have to do the root canal you look like a winner. If you have to do a root canal, and you didn't tell the patient about this possibility, then you will look like a goat. Have the unpredictable work to your advantage. Don't try to work calcification miracles - your patients will lose their trust in you if they have problems with a filling that you just placed.

I tell all of my patients who exhibit deep cavities of the possibility for endodontic therapy. If I have any doubt about the future prognosis of the pulp, I will commence with root canal treatment. I can perform a molar root canal in less than 45 minutes. It is a safe and beneficial service for your patients. Learn to perform it. Your income will benefit tremendously. Your patients will appreciate the comfort.

Liners such as Hemaseal plus Ionoseal can work at times so long as you have at least 1 mm of dentin left. Otherwise, root canal!

It does not take long to learn how to perform endodontics. All you need is a positive attitude and a desire to learn. The only root canals I refer are lower second molars with extremely curved roots and re-treatment of another practitioner's previous failure. I will also refer lower apicoectomies/retrogrades. I don't like to work around the canal. Otherwise, I do all of my endodontics, including upper apicoectomies, hemisections, and root amputations.

In order to become proficient at endodontics you must learn the anatomy of root morphology of all of the teeth that you want to treat. Of course, an adequate periapical X-ray is your best teacher. Don't cone-cut your x-rays...use proper angulation. Pre-plan your therapy by studying the pre-op X-ray of the tooth in question. Evaluate the curvature of the roots and the number of canals. Sometimes it is necessary to get different views in order to be able to evaluate all factors.

NEVER commence therapy of the pulp without studying the pre-op radiograph.

Once you have decided to proceed with root canal therapy, your most important step is to adequately and completely remove all decay from the tooth. Judge the restorability of the tooth before you spend time on the root canal. Once you have decided that your tooth is restorable and your margins are free of caries, find the pulp chamber, open it up and locate the canals. Follow the basics of anatomy when locating the canals. Use a #8 file to enter the canal and begin biomechanical preparation. Also, use your endo explorer and/or the #8 file to locate any accessory canals. Once you have freed the contents of the canals with the #8 file (or Pathfinders), proceed with the #10 and #20 file and take your length X-ray. Use some RC Prep to help open the canals. Make sure that you have used a reference point for your length. It is a good idea to flatten the reference point (reduce the cusp) in order to give you an easier plateau for judging the place of your rubber stopper. I usually find one reference point for all canals. <u>The reference point is extremely important!!!</u>

Once you have established the proper length, turn the procedure over to your rotaries. I use Protaper files.

Biomechanical preparation is fairly easy once your access into the canals has been established. Sometimes it may be easier to actually use the first rotary file (S1) to access calcified or stuck canals, instead of hand files. Go slowly!

Don't be afraid to remove extra enamel and tooth tissue to help you gain entry and access. This is especially true for the <u>mesials of the lower molars</u>...remove enough facial and lingual tooth tissue to give you enough access and visibility.

To complete preparation of the canals, go through your sequence and make sure that you use gentle finger pressure and NEVER, EVER force files down canals. I also use RC Prep and my assistant rinses the tooth with my PB during preparation with each and every file. The PB disinfects and acts as a lubricant also.

Don't be in a rush to get to the next file. Use each file until you feel it practically floating in the canal. Then proceed to the next size, and so on. I also like to use a #10 file at end of my preparation to **detangle any left-over debris at the apex** . I do this by gently pushing this file slightly past and through the apical foramen. I am not afraid to do this because I will not "blow-out" the apex. I only use a few light strokes and the size 10 is not big enough to cause any damage. Making sure that my apex is clean ensures that I do not leave any fostering bacteria that can habitate this location and come back to cause a civil unrest in a few years.

Always pay attention to the rubber stopper, and therefore the length of your file. During the up and down motion of the filing, the stopper can move and your length can be affected. **Stop and double check the position of your stopper often. Take the file out and remeasure it**. Double-check your reference point. It does not take long to do this. Losing your length can be detrimental to success. Using a file shorter than the required length will cause you to ledge the canal. Once you do this it may be impossible to re-establish your length. Use an <u>endodontic measuring block</u> when measuring your files. **Maintain your working length!!!**

One of the most important decisions that you will have to make while performing endodontics is the determination of the file size that you will end your preparation with. Although this varies according to the canal's size, shape and anatomy, you should be able to assess your final file size by evaluating the pre-op x-ray. Of course, once you start to feel the file "sticking" to the sides of the canal you should be contemplating your conclusion of preparation. The main exception to this dental school philosophy is for calcified canals. Here are a few other helpful suggestions:

1. Mesial canals of lower molars usually require a preparation to size F2. I have never taken a mesial canal on these teeth past a size F3. If the curvature is pronounced and/or the tooth is very thin I will stop at F1. It is helpful to take different angled x-rays, from mesial to distal, in order to check for accessory canals and differences in length of the facial and lingual canals (it is rare to find differences in length, however). Angled views will also help you to see whether the distal may have accessory canals.

2. Distal canals of lower molars usually require at least a size F3 preparation and many times I will switch back to regular files (using a M4 handpiece) and find myself at 60. Distals can often have 2 canals that converge and filing them past a 50 may be necessary. Most of the time you will file to a size 60. Double check accessory canals!!!

3. Lower premolars usually require at least a size F3 or maybe back to regular files around 50. One canal is the norm.

4. Upper premolars normally have two roots with slight distal curvature. Even with two canals, I like to file these teeth to a size F3, unless the curvature is pronounced. It is very important to take different views with your x-rays in order to determine any differences in length of your canals. Sometimes these teeth have a lingual canal which is of shorter length than the facial, and vice versa. I take a normal Periapical (bisected angle view) of the tooth as well as a mesial to disto-lingual view. Using the old SLOB rule, I know that the canal which moved to the distal on the x-ray is the facial canal. Increase the exposure time a little when taking this x-ray. Double check the length of each canal (make sure you have a file in each canal...hah, hah). Sometimes it is easy to miss the lingual canal during access opening because this guy likes to hide right under the lingual cusp tip. Make sure you widen your

access opening so that you can get to it. If they have one root, I switch to regular files and end up around 55.

5. Upper molars have three canals and they normally vary in length. Your length x-ray should have 3 canals with 3 different files showing 3 different lengths. Double check the mesio-facial canal for accessories. I normally take the palatal canal to a size 60 or larger. With the facials I rarely go past a size F3. If they are curved, I end with a F2.

6. Upper anteriors normally range from a size 60 to even as high as 90 or 100. Lower incisors usually are prepared to a size 40.

7. Always use sharp files. Discard bald files. Your first 2 rotary files should be discarded after each use but you can try to get one sterilization cycle from your bigger rotaries.

Once my biomechanical preparation is completed, and I feel confident that I have gained adequate access for my points, I begin to custom fit and size all of the points at once. I keep the canals wet so that the points slide down easily. I purchase only the following sized gutta perchas in my arsenal: F1-F4, 50, 55, 60, 70

Of course, I establish tug-back and verify the fit with an x-ray. Always!!!

Once everything fits to my standards, I redip the points in my PB solution and I dry the canals. My final fill is done by carrying MTA or Tubliseal sealer down the canals with a lentulo spiral. It is not necessary to fit the spiral all the way to the apex. Once you place the points, the sealer will extrude down to the apex. I cut my points, and then I use the Touch'N Heat to melt the coronal part of the points.

It does not matter what type of obturation technique you use as long as your preparation was properly performed.

The success of your endodontics will NOT be based on a good looking fill. Success starts with adequate and complete biomechanical preparation along with disinfection of bacteria. The gutta percha and the sealer will not destroy or fixate left-over bacteria. All pulp contents must be cleaned out and the walls of the preparation must be smooth like glass. Debris or any pulp contents left behind can cause future failure. The sealer and gutta percha are placed to help seal and fill the void in order to prevent leakage from above (coronal part), laterally, and only minimally from inside the canal. They are basically there to guard and insure against any bacterial re-activation. Complete preparation and removal of contents renders the sealing part, more or less, as an adjunctive aspect. The best filled root canal will fail if the biomechanical preparation was hurried, minimal, or incomplete. The worst filled root canal will still be successful, if the canals were cleaned completely.

After you have completed the root canal you must take into account the final restoration. Leaving temporaries on for too long (more than a week) can result in microleakage and failure. **Most endodontic failures occur because of poor fitting restorations that allow microleakage from the mouth into the pulp chamber and down around the root canal sealer.** Bacteria will seep around gutta percha like a hot knife through butter. As they reach the apex, guess what happens? Do everything possible to place a good fitting core and crown as soon as possible.

Preferably, the same day!

I don't use thermofilling techniques. I do not use these techniques because I like to be able to check my fit prior to final sealing. <u>Thermofillers are great if you have an ideal situation, but this is far from reality in the clinic. Pre-fitting cones is often a necessity.</u> I also don't feel that thermofillers save me that much time.

I see a lot of specialists and general dentists performing ten-visit root canals. Over the years, I have learned that **99% of endodontic procedures should be completed on the same visit.** The only exception to this rule is a chronic or acute infection which exhibits drainage. Even if the patient shows up at my office with a throbbing toothache, I will complete and seal the root canal without hesitation, unless I see and smell "gunk." If you stick an absorbent point into the canal, after your preparation is completed, and you get the old, putrid, foul smell you may want to wait seven or 10 days. Otherwise, seal the puppy!!! Two-visit root canals allow for bacterial colonization and negative patient marketing. Nobody wants to come to your office for two root canal visits for one tooth, except the anaerobic germs.

To increase the success of your endodontic procedures, prescribe strong antibiotics and pain meds. My basic antibiotic is still Amoxicillin. I dispense it for all root canals post-op, as well as pre-op. It is great to be able to have a root canal patient start taking Amoxicillin beginning 2 days pre-op. The tooth and the bone will be calm and the recovery will be speedy. I routinely use Augmentin (875 mg., tid x 7 days) for more severe infections. If these first two are not enough to do the job, I add Flagyl (250 mg. tid x 5 days) to the regimen (with careful consideration to patient response and side-effects). This may only be necessary once in a great while, but the combination works great for anaerobic annihilation. Sometimes I will also use Doxycycline or Erythromycin for upper teeth and/or teeth with periodontal involvement. The Doxy is great for periodontal bacteria and the Erythromycin works wonders for any apical infections encroaching the sinus. Obviously for patients allergic to Penicillin, you cannot prescribe Amoxicillin so switch to Z-Pak 7 day (Azithromycin).

I have one more drug that I call "Wonder-Drug:" **Prednisone.** This corticosteroid, prescribed in 5 mg tablets works miracles for calming down "hot" teeth and preventing the midnight call from today's last root canal patient. I prescribe this medication for all of my root canals, periodontal surgeries, extractions, and sometimes prosthodontic procedures. Prednisone 5 mg tid x 5 days. You will be known as Dr. Miracle.

The last prescription that I give my patients is for pain meds. I try to stick to T3 or Norco 5/325. They can take 1 or even 2 tabs every 4 hrs. for 3 days. Make sure they sign the Narcotic Counseling Forms.

STRIVE FOR EXCELLENCE, NOT PERFECTION

DONATE

ENCOURAGE HOPE

REMEMBER NAMES

LEARN CPR, YEARLY

CHAPTER 30
CORES/BUILD-UPS

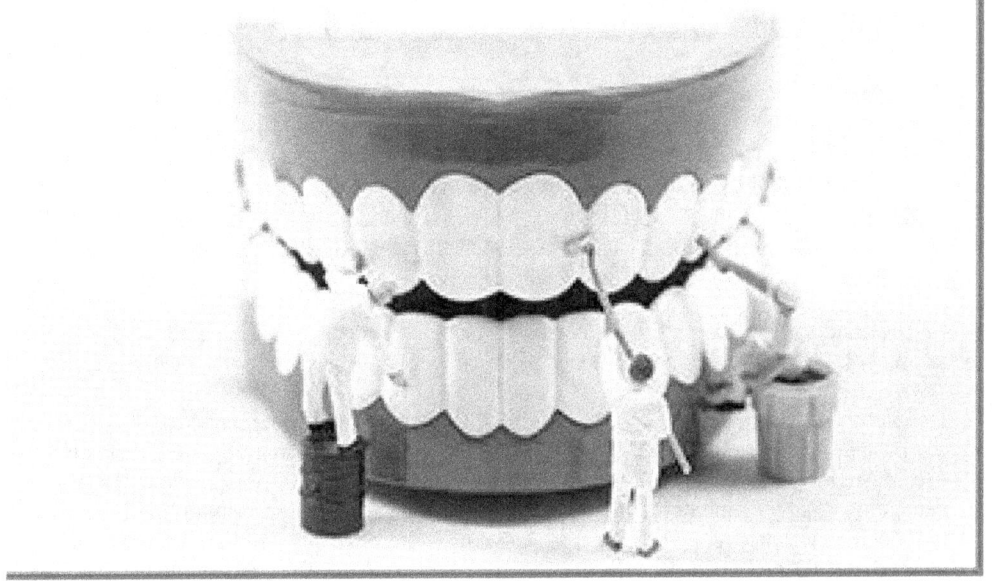

A lot has changed in recent years in regard to bonding agents and cores. Today's bonding agents are making post systems a thing of the past. Some of the latest research show that when trying to break or loosen a bonded core, most teeth will fracture and break at other points of their anatomy other than at the bonded core.

Before doing a core, re-evaluate the status of your pulp and/or root canal seal. Take the appropriate steps if endo therapy is required, or if the root canal seal is inadequate.

Do not core until you are certain that the root canal is adequate!!!!!!!!!!!!!!!!!!!!

A core build-up is one of your most profitable procedures. It should not take longer than 15 minutes. <u>I perform core build-ups for all of my crown preparations, whether or not the tooth has been treated endodontically</u>. I still use posts routinely and for the following circumstances:

1. Complete loss of anatomy (including molars).
2. Anteriors and premolars.

It is rare that I place a post in a molar tooth, unless I am working on the Incredible Hulk, and there is very little anatomy left. There is nothing wrong with placing a post, if the endo is perfect. Don't overlook the advantages of the extra strength and retention that the post gives the tooth and the core. **I like to place posts in all of my premolars and anteriors** because I believe that it helps to compensate for possible future mid-root fractures. Anteriors take a lot of lateral loads. A post that is of adequate length and properly bonded to the cementum of the root reinforces the root system and gives it additional strength. I don't believe research that states teeth get weakened when posts are used. If the post is properly bonded into the root how can it weaken it?

Here is the simple process of doing a core, including post placement:

1. Prep canal with Peezo-Reamer (5 mm. short of apex). **Remove all gutta percha and attain clean canal walls**. Use plenty of alcohol on the Peezo-Reamer to help remove the eugenol and sealer. Finish with the appropriate Para-Post Drills. It is very important to clean the root free of any eugenol by using alcohol on the reamers and drills. Soak your root with alcohol! If not placing a post you must still remove at least 2 mm. of gutta percha down and into each canals. There must be no gutta percha or sealer anywhere in the pulp chamber or showing from the canals.

2. Fit post and trim to length (check occlusion to make sure that you have allowed plenty of clearance). Make sure you have attained as much length as possible for the post.

3. Double check caries removal. Clean the tooth with alcoholed microbrushes, etch, and dry tooth/canal. Don't forget to stick air-water syringe down in the canal to get the debris out (or use an irrigant syringe). Use absorbent points to dry canal thoroughly. Make sure that you are cementing against cementum and not gutta percha. I see so many posts failing because the gutta percha was not removed properly. Any core system will function for a lifetime, as long as you have cleaned the dentin and cementum free of any eugenol and other material.

   Core materials do not fail because they are weak. They fail because of improper placement and inadequate tooth preparation/cleansing.

4. Seal any canals that are not receiving posts with a Glass Ionomer cement (RMGI-Kerr). Just make sure that you are getting it at least 2 mm. down into the canal spaces so that you get a good seal and prevent any leakage. Finish these cores with composite.

5. Optibond

6. Syringe RMGI or core material into canal and around canal entry. Place post down canal and make sure it is seated all the way down. Also make sure that it does not get extruded back out by the hydrostatic pressure of the cement.. The post will push the core material down into the canal, as long as you have placed enough of it into the canal opening to begin with. This helps to create a complete, tight post-system that is as strong as a custom post. It is also bonded into the cementum of the root system.

You can use your favorite core material as the cement for the post and final core material. I like to use RMGI as my post cement but then I use Omnichroma to finish the core. Right after seating the post, I bulk fill and use my finger (with a little Optibond on it) to push the material into the tooth and around the post. I like knowing that my RMGI (glass ionomer) is extruding and sealing my cementum and dentin. I like having a glass ionomer on cementum or dentin as it has good seal properties down there. My Omnichroma is strong core material.

For anterior teeth and premolars you may want to use Fiber Posts due to cosmetic reasons. I normally still use metal posts because the Omnichroma Blocker hides the metal well. Recently, I have been leaning towards using Fiber Posts with the RelyX cement.

When doing cores on vital teeth I still use composite. With the latest dentinal bonding agents I feel that the composite makes a great core for a vital tooth. Don't be afraid to etch the dentin and the enamel. Seal the dentinal tubules and make sure that you used your PB solution to thoroughly disinfect the tooth. Also, remember to cure the composite slowly. For most small to medium vital cores all you need is a flowable. You don't have to worry about compressive strength, since your main goal is to seal the tooth and eliminate undercuts. Do the core before any marginal preparation so that you have no bleeding. You do not want blood or astringents ruining your core. Follow the same dentinal sealing procedures as described in Chapter 28.

I always use a matrix, along with adequate isolation. For vital teeth, even when I have adequate tooth anatomy left, I still perform a composite core but I do NOT bill insurance or patient for it. **A broken down tooth, without endo, is made stronger and more retentive through a core build-up**. The impression is made simpler, undercuts are removed, margins are easier to detect, the temporary fits better, and final crown seating is simplified. Your lab person will love you and the core also helps to decrease post-op sensitivity.

EVERYONE HAS A CHOICE IN LIFE

CHAPTER 31
CROWNS/PROSTHETICS

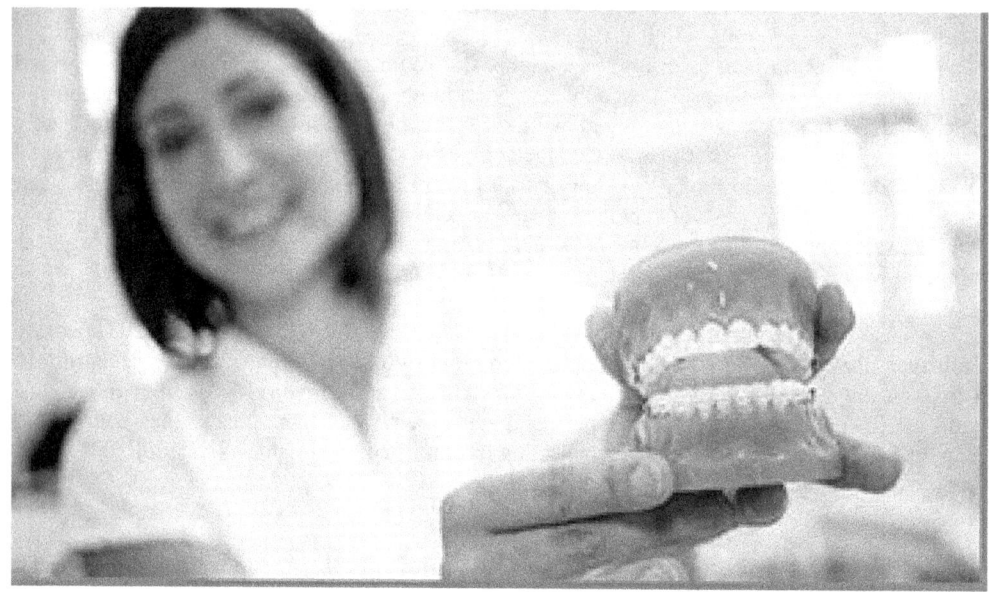

All of your crown and prosthetic procedures should start with careful evaluation of the occlusion. The longevity and fit of your prosthodontic work will depend largely on the patient's occlusion. It will also depend on the procedures that you follow and the impression techniques that you use. Of course, the periodontium has to be healthy and the vitality and/or endodontic state must be carefully evaluated.

To fabricate a well-fitting and esthetic crown your procedure depends on proper preparation and perfect impression techniques. The type of impression and tray that you will use should be determined at the onset of your appointment. Preferably, it should be determined during your treatment planning and pre-op preparation, for all cases involving multiple units.

Although I have been using Itero for the past 10 years, the following are simple basics. If you do not have a digital scanner then follow these protocols. The first thing you must do is to pick the appropriate tray. For all single units I use disposable plastic bite trays. I like to use the largest sizes available in order to get the most teeth impresssed for good occlusal analysis and insurance against any distortion. I try to pick up the cuspids in all of my impressions. Cuspid guidance is important and your impression must allow for its duplication. The only time that I use full arch trays for single units is when I have a larger than normal tooth and I can sense that the tooth will hit the sides of the tray upon biting. You can usually tell that this has happened when you see parts of the tray showing through your impression close to the preparation, especially the sides of the tray. These drag marks indicate distortion. Use full arch trays if this happens or the crown will not fit.

Obviously if I am doing more than 2 units I have to use a full-arch tray. When using full arch trays try to use the most rigid trays available. Custom made trays are not necessary for 2 to 3 units, as there are plenty of acceptable rigid trays on the market. Just make sure that they have ample holes for retention and material venting. Some trays lack holes on the lingual aspects. Buy trays that have holes or you must cut into the tray to create the holes. Always use as much adhesive on the trays as possible. You can never have enough adhesive or holes for retention!!! You do NOT want your impression material pulling away from the tray. For more than 3 units, you should consider using custom trays.

Visualize the tray in the patient's mouth. If the tray is not going down into the vestibule easily without hitting a few teeth, or it does not fit all the way down over the cervicals, it is too small. It is much better to use a larger tray than a smaller one. You can also use a little heat to bend and re-shape the tray. Avoid distortion upon biting by making sure that the tray sits passively! **Any pressure or distortion on the tray will distort the impression**. Do not be afraid to use a full arch tray when you feel that the triple-tray is too small for your patient.

Before you begin preparation don't forget to take a hard-body impression of the arch or quadrant - this is the **preliminary impression** which will be used to make the temporary. I use Monophase for this. You can also use thermal buttons if you like but I have found them to be inaccurate and cumbersome. If the tooth is broken down make sure that you build it back up with Cavit, DuoTemp, core material, or even ortho wax before you take your preliminary impression. Remember that you will use this anatomy as your guide when making the temporary.

When doing multiple units you should take a full arch preliminary impression if the teeth are anatomically correct. If the multiple units are not anatomically sound you will obviously need to do a lab wax-up and make temporaries before you start. When doing bridges you will definitely have to prefabricate your temporaries. Biotemps are the simplest solution.

Now that your preliminary impression has been taken, you are ready for the preparation. Once you have determined that the crown margins do not require periodontal lengthening, the preparation should proceed without difficulty. Of course, you have checked the periodontal pocketing depths and made sure that the tissue is healthy. All periodontal treatment should be completed before the crown preparation, except for slightly hyperplastic tissue reduction, which can be reduced during your preparation.

When preparing your crown, do not worship tooth structure. **Inadequate reduction leads to lab problems and prehistoric results**. Review the anatomy of the tooth and take into account furcations and margin depths. Make sure that you maintain steady hand posture and appropriate draw. All preparations are done with counterclockwise movement of the handpiece around the tooth. Once the occlusal table has been cleared and you have plenty of room, start the axial aspects of the preps. Begin on the occlusal half and work your way down and around. If you try to start working on your cervical margin areas first you may end up creating undercuts.

Don't bend and change the head of the handpiece in order to create your margins. Proper marginal definition will be a result of counter- clockwise rotation of your handpiece being held in the appropriate draw position. Don't alter the five degree rule of draw. Let your margins form as you remove enamel and dentin from the axial walls.

General rule for amount of reduction:

- 1.0 mm. for gold
- 1.5 - 2.0 mm. for all-porcelain
- 2.0 - 2.5 mm. for occlusal and incisal

Use tracer cuts as guides!!!

Remember that shade guides are 4 mm. thick. Your lab cannot duplicate these shades if you do not give them ample reduction.

Sometimes you have to remove gum tissue in order to prepare your margins. Hyperplastic tissue must be removed in order to ensure proper fit and adaptation. Buy a Laser! When working in the anterior region you should wait two weeks before final impression, if you have removed more than 1mm. of gum tissue and you are not comfortable with how the gums will heal. Future exposed metal margins, or exposed root surfaces, can lead to remakes and unhappy patients. Again, healthy periodontium before successful restorative!!!

It is a good idea to pick one type of margin preparation and use this for most of your preparations. I like the chamfer style. I use it for my posterior preparations as well as my anterior. The only variation in design is that I reduce a little more tooth structure for porcelain crowns than for gold. For all-ceramic crowns I will vary my preparation to more of a deeper chamfer. I use a 1 1/2 mm. diameter diamond for my Zirconia crowns. It does not matter which brand of diamond you decide to use. Pick the appropriate diameter according to how much reduction you want...then use the diamond as a tracer and as your main bur. Of course, for occlusal reduction, you should use a flame or football shaped diamond. Try to stay with the same type of bur! You should not need more than a football diamond and a chamfer diamond for all of your preparations.

WHEN REDUCING FOLLOW THE CONTOUR OF THE TOOTH!

One of the most important parts of preparing your tooth is to make sure that you visualize all aspects of your margins. This means that you must see the proximal aspects of your finish. This can become difficult when you have broken cusps or deep decayed tooth anatomy that has been covered over by gum tissue. It is important to REDUCE all hyperplastic gingiva in order to clearly define your margins. You want to achieve less than 3 mm of pocket depth and clear visualization of your margins. Reduce the tissue vertically and then "pull" the margin away from the tooth by reducing the internal aspect of the gingiva so that you don't have to use cord. At times, broken down teeth will hide the cervico-proximal extension of the margins. I routinely use my Laser to remove gum tissue and control hemostasis. Get in the habit of making friends with your laser.

Once you have finished your preparation, and you can clearly and completely visualize your margins, you are ready to proceed with the impression. This is the most important part of all of your hard work. Your entire outcome depends on this step.

In order to achieve a great impression you must also **control bleeding spots and have a clean tooth**. Again, your Laser and 1:50,000 Xylocaine should be enough armament for this Battle of the Bulge. If any bleeding remains, after using the laser, you can simply use Astringedent (Ultradent Co) syringe tips. The Ultradent syringe tips (Luer-Lock tips) are cotton tipped syringes that you fill with Astringedent. The Ultradent syringe tips are exceptionally easy to use. Squeeze and go!!! For anteriors, use the clear Astringent so that you don't get discoloration of the tooth. Do NOT "moat" around the gingival with these by using circular swiping motions. The only way to stop bleeding is to use vertical pressure on the arteriole that is bleeding. If you go around in circles you will open up more bleeding spots. Vertical, specific and spot controlled pressure only. You can also use Traxodent with pressure caps to stop bleeding.

Once the bleeding is controlled, I thoroughly clean the tooth with my PB mixture. If I did not reduce enough tissue with the laser I either go back to reducing more tissue or I will pack cord into the gum. The size of the cord depends on the depth of the pocketing left and the amount of gingivectomy that you have performed. Again, your goal is to reduce the tissue so that you have an "ideal" 3 mm of pocket left and horizontal separation of tissue away from margins. If you did not achieve this then you can place a size (0) cord to separate the tissue away from the tooth. Once the cord is tightly packed in the gums I rinse with a little Astringedent and let it sit for 60 seconds. Then, I completely rinse all hemostatic agent from the cord and tooth. **Leaving the agent on for longer than 2 minutes will cause rebound bleeding and post-op sensitivity, due to the caustic effect of the astringent**. After the agent is rinsed, I wait at least 2 more minutes and then I wet the cord and remove it. Never take the cord out unless you wet it with water. Taking out a dry cord will pull the coagulated particles away from the vessels and cause rebound bleeding.

If there is any rebound bleeding after cord removal, I am forced into using more Astringdent around the area, and maybe even re-packing cord. This should not be necessary in most crown procedures, if you have taken all of the previous procedures seriously and non-hastily. More epinephrine is also helpful.

Don't forget to go back and <u>thoroughly clean the tooth free of any debris with the PB</u>. You want to take an impression of the tooth, not of coagulated particles.

Clean tooth, will travel!!!

Before you take your impression, you should consider whether your dentin is still sealed from the previous core placement that you have done, if you are working on a vital tooth. Most likely you have removed the bond layer during your marginal preparation and you may want to go back and reseal. Clean with PB, etch, and place more Hemaseal.

Before impressing, you should also consider what has happened in the sulcular area. You most probably have trapped debris and resins from your preparation and core placement. Clean the sulcus!!! Use the PB and scrub it clean.

Note: I cannot stress how important it is to make sure that all of the teeth are clean and free of any debris before you take any impressions. This is very important, especially when doing large cases. If you are going to take any full arch impression, get your patient out of the chair and brush their teeth with a regular toothbrush. Get ALL of the teeth as clean as a whistle. Polish the teeth, if you have to. Just get them clean!!! You don't want anything being picked up in the impression that can lead to distortion. This is also true for all of your alginates and your denture and partial impressions.

Once everything is up to par, take your final impression using your light and heavy body material.

When pulling the impression out have the patient close their lips together and blow out the tray, instead of opening their mouth or tugging on the impression. This helps to prevent distortion. <u>You should get in the habit of doing this for all of your impression procedures</u>, including alginates. Don't play teeter-totter with your trays - this will lead to distortion. If the patient cannot close their lips together and blow the tray out, use the air-water syringe and blow air and water around the buccal extensions. This will loosen the tray and make it easier to take out.

One of my dental school mentors was a dental product researcher. His advice in regard to picking the best impression material was simple: you can use any material you desire as long as you learn how to use it correctly. I know practitioners who use alginate for multiple bridge procedures and achieve text-book results. I also know practitioners who use Impregum and achieve sub-standard results. It is not the material. It is the technique. Currently I use Impregum for some of my deep/long margin preps, implant and multiple unit work ….but the Itero does 99% of my work!

I hear many of my colleagues complaining about their lab person's workmanship and crown fit. I usually tell them the same thing: **it's not your lab!!!...it's your technique**. When a crown does not fit, or the occlusion is too high, it is usually not your lab's fault. It is your fault, if the crown looks good on the die!!!

The main reason for a poorly fitting crown is BAD impression technique.

Temporization is usually the next step, before the final impression is taken. I used to wait until after taking the impression to make the temporary. With today's temporary materials and dentinal sealing procedures I like to use the preliminary impression as a mold for the temporary. An excellent fitting provisional is easy to make.

Poorly fitting temporaries lead to frustration during the cementation appointment.

Bad temporary margins cause gingival irritation and hyperplasia, which results in extra periodontal work during the cementation appointment.

Low occlusal stops in the temporary lead to more bite, bite, grind, grind steps at the final appointment.

Don't be in a rush to finish the temporary and get the patient out the door. **A properly fitted temporary results in a quick and efficient final appointment.**

There are basically 2 ways to make temporaries:

1. Use the preliminary impression.
2. Lab fabricated (Biotemps)

Try to use option 2 every time.

I use Integrity for all my temporaries.
If my assistant forgets to take a preliminary impression then I have 2 choices:

1. make the temporary by hand using Jet. If I have to make the temporary by hand (happens once every 5 years) I mix a ball of Jet to doughy consistency and place it on the preparation slowly, while molding it on the buccal and lingual. As it begins to set, I have the patient bite down into it. I trim it with scissors before it hardens and place it back on the prep for one or two more bites. Sometimes these temporaries have to be relined. If you have to reline you must grind out the entire internal aspect before you reline, otherwise your temporary will not fit back down over the tooth properly. Do this extra step to make sure that your margins fit properly.
2. Take ortho wax or DuoTemp and rebuild the tooth, then take the preliminary impression.

I use Jet for all of my multiple unit work because my lab provides Biotemps for my big cases which need to be relined with Jet.

When I use the preliminary impression, I allow the Integrity 1 1/2 minutes to set in the mouth. Then, I remove it and let it harden on the counter. I wait another 60 seconds, remove it from the impression, and analyze the margins. If there is any discrepancy I redo it. Don't forget to polish the temporary with your buff wheel before cementing it. You don't want your patient pulling it out because it feels rough.

After you complete the temporary, go back in the mouth and check for any stray temporary material. This stuff can practically become invisible at times. Take a scaler and feel around all of the teeth to **make sure that you don't have any Integrity left on any teeth.** Also check the opposing quadrant. Clean all the teeth!!!

To cement your temporaries use Temp-Bond. Don't forget to remove excess cement from the margins with floss and your explorer. Excess cement will lead to irritation and bleeding. Use

Vaseline on the temp and adjacent teeth before temporarily cementing so that your clean up is made easier.

When the crown comes back from the lab you should have a fast and efficient appointment to seat it. A properly fabricated crown should seat in under 10 minutes. If it does not consider the following "clinical audit" and find the common faults:

1. **Using the wrong tray (tray too small).**
2. **Bleeding gums.**
3. **Lousy preparation.**
4. **Poor temporization.**

Before you pick up the phone and decide to scream at your lab, step back funky cat. Re-evaluate your margins, your occlusion, and your impression technique. If you are having doubts about your lab, get in the habit of keeping a second set of duplicate models/dies in your office. This is easy to do if you pour your own dies, which you should. These can be your soft-tissue dies or *check dies*. Many labs perform this extra step, because they use these duplicate models when making the final crown adjustments. When the crown comes back from the lab try the crown on your *check* model. If it does not fit, maybe you can blame the lab. But first, try to adjust and make the crown fit on these models, if the lab has not already done so. Consider this your pre-fitting appointment before the patient arrives. Use Occlude Spray, or food coloring, to mark the dies and see where there may be tight areas (coloring will be removed off of the die where the crown is tight). If the crown does not fit, then maybe the lab altered your dies. Usually, the only way they can alter dies is to cut margins short. To guard against shortened margins, pencil your margin lines and place Crazy Glue over them before the lab begins the work. This will seal the mark and make it hard for your lab to change the margin.

If the crown fits on the models, but it does not go down on the tooth, after attempting to adjust it, your impression was distorted. Possible reasons include:

1. Your tray was small. It most likely hit a large bony vestibule or it was too small for the size of the tooth being impressed.

2. You believed the manufacturer of your impression material when they told you that you can use the "hydrophilic" material even if you have bleeding. Think about that for a moment. Can your impression material really "suck-up" blood and debris? No way! You need a clean tooth and complete hemostasis, otherwise your impression will distort.

Your final cementation appointment should be an easy and fast procedure, once you have followed all of the above steps. After you remove the temporary you should notice practically no bleeding. Always numb your patient, especially for vital teeth preparations. Clean the tooth thoroughly with the PB solution. Try not to get too aggressive around the gingival area. **If there is any bleeding you must control it by cord-packing and/or using your favorite astringent. There must be absolutely no bleeding and you must have a very clean tooth, including the sulcus.**

Seat the crown on the preparation and check the contacts with floss. This should be your first step. Tight contacts will not allow your crown to seat down all the way. **After the contacts are adjusted, take at least 2 bitewing x-rays to evaluate your subgingival margin fit.** For anteriors, make sure that the P.A. is properly angled to show the interproximal area without distortion.

Never cement a crown without checking the bitewing and/or P.A.!

Adjust the occlusion while the x-ray is being developed. Also, check the marginal adaptation on the buccal and lingual. If the bitewings show a good fit, you are ready to cement the crown, as long as the patient is happy with the occlusion, the shade, and the overall fit.

Never cement crowns, especially anteriors, without approval from the patient!!!

At the sake of being redundant: if there is any gingival bleeding, you must take out the laser or pack cord and control the blood. Don't seat your crown, unless the tooth is completely clean and the gums are totally healthy. Cementing the crown over a dirty preparation will decrease the longevity of your tooth and cause recurrent decay. It will also decrease the bond strength of your cement and cause pulpitis on vital teeth. If there has been any gingival hyperplasia, you must laser this tissue before you seat the crown. Again, use your laser! Don't get into the philosophy that your cement will extrude the gums out of the way as you seat the crown down. It won't! You must have a clean, visible environment without any element interfering with your margins and your tooth upon final seating. Don't trap red blood cells under your crown. If your temporary fit well, you should not have too much to worry about. <u>Aren't you glad you spend enough time making a great fitting temporary?</u>

CLEAN TOOTH, HEALTHY GUMS - WILL TRAVEL!!!

I use Speedcem for all my work since I mainly do Zirconias. For veneers, I use Nexxus.
My crown seat steps are simple:

1. Prepare crown with Monobond
2. Place Vaseline on outside of crown
3. Place Vaseline on interproximal areas of adjacent teeth paying careful attention to not touch the prep. If doing a bridge I coat all outside areas of bridge with Vaseline and wrap Floss in the embrasure areas
4. Seat Crown with Speedcem and have patient bite down.
5. "Wave" Cure the cement around the buccal margins by sweeping for 2-3 seconds with the curing light while patient is biting. You are trying to "fix" the crown into position and also trying to start the curing of the cement around the margins
6. Do the same "Wave" on the lingual and then….
7. Remove the tacky cement with scaler
8. Have assistant hold crown with finger while flossing interproximal
9. Cure completely for 1 minute
10. Scale remaining cement.

Keep a saliva ejector in the vestibule, along with cotton rolls, to minimize saliva contamination.

Multiple unit prosthetics is an extension of your single unit procedures. The main difference is more pre-planning and a more work. If you are going to be restoring any of your patients with fixed bridges that are bigger than 4 units I would highly recommend that you seek the expertise and direction of a prosthodontist. Do not get in the habit of doing large cases at the beginning of your career. Prosthodontics requires much more clinical experience and knowledge than dental school has provided you with. Refer all of your large and difficult cases to a prosthodontist. Follow through with the patient's progress and learn from the specialist during this process. Learn to diagnose and plan the larger cases properly. Don't jump into them without more education. **You need to learn how to evaluate occlusions and case designs. Dental school knowledge is not enough!!!**

I recently had a patient come to my office who had just spent $14000 at another office for fixed bridges. She complained of poor fit, lousy esthetics, and inability to chew properly. After a complete work-up, including mounted study models, I realized that she had a legitimate problem. The previous dentist had placed two four unit bridges on the upper right and left, and one six unit bridge on the lower left. The occlusion was off, the shades did not match, and the overall function was improper. He had to give the patient a refund.

Doing three unit bridges is basically a fairly easy procedure that any young practitioner can accomplish with excellent results. I like to fabricate preliminary temporaries for all of my bridges. Any lab can do this for you.

LET YOUR LAB DO IT (Biotemp from Glidewell), but if you want to save lab cost, follow these steps:

1. Double pour all models.
2. Use the second models to do preparations of the abutments; use your regular diamonds and prepare the teeth **just as though you were doing your final preparations, except prepare with as minimal reduction as possible**. Do not over-reduce because it will result in poor fit if your preparations don't match the reduction. Mimic your reduction into gingival areas, in order to get adequate coverage.
3. Use the first models as study and wax models. Wax-in the pontic teeth, or use denture teeth, to fill in the edentulous area. Mount them!!!
4. Take an alginate of the completed waxed study model from step 3. Pour it in stone. Make a vacuum formed shell over this poured model. You can use this shell intraorally to make your temporary, OR...
5. After pouring the model in step 4, be careful and save the alginate impression. Remove it from the model and fill the abutment and pontic teeth with the temporary material. It helps to have some *vent* holes. Use Jet because when you get to the mouth it will give you good working time.
6. Place the filled alginate over the second, prepared models from step 2.
7. Let completely set.

8. Remove the set temporary bridge and trim margins. Unfortunately the models from step 2 will be destroyed, so get in the habit of having extra copies of all of your models (double pour your alginates).
9. Trim occlusion.
10. <u>If you are replacing an existing bridge this entire sequence can be eliminated.</u> Simply take an intraoral impression using your regular impression material (quadrant tray is adequate as long as it can cover three unprepared teeth) before you cut off the old bridge.

<u>If you are placing an initial bridge</u> in the posterior and there are edentulous areas, you should be fine without a temporary bridge so long as your lab completes the bridge within 2 weeks. If patient wants to see what it will look like, order a Biotemp from Glidewell.

<u>Back to the regular way:</u> after your bridge abutments are prepared intraorally you simply try in the indirect temporary bridge that you have fabricated. If it fits closely, all you have to do is reline it with temporary material of the same kind. Use Jet. You have saved a lot of chair time and guaranteed a great fit. Just be careful about relining it. You won't have more than one opportunity for a good reline. Second and third relines will be difficult, unless you completely relieve the internal aspects in order to make the temporary fit passively over the abutments.
If the temporary does not fit, even after adjustments, you still have your vacuum-formed shells that you can use. That's why you should always go through the effort of making these shells. You can also use these type of shells as guides to show clearance for adequate porcelain thickness when preparing anterior teeth.

When seating your multiple unit prosthetics, occlusion is very critical. Sometimes the articulating paper does not adequately mark your contacts and you may get frustrated trying to figure out if the crown or bridge fits properly. This usually happens when the bridge is too high or when there is saliva on the porcelain. First, get yourself a landmark without the bridge in place. Use whatever occlusal stops you can see easily as reference landmarks. Let's say I am doing a posterior bridge. Before placing any posterior prosthesis in the mouth I always check the anterior stops. After I put the crown or bridge in the mouth I recheck the anterior contacts again. If they don't touch (open occlusion) I know that I need to do some bite, bite, grind, grind. Get the occlusion into harmony or your work will fail. This suggestion is also useful when seating single units. Also, use folded gauze or cotton rolls to dry the occlusals of the restorations. Have the patient bite into the gauze or cotton roll. If the patient does not bite there may still be moisture on the occlusal surfaces. **Dry the teeth!!!**

On the other side of midnight, make sure that the occlusion is not too light. Use shimstock to make sure that you have adequate contacts. Crowns will hypererupt into occlusion, but bridges may not! I actually instruct my laboratory to leave my crowns shy of occlusion because I know that the tooth will erupt into occlusion in a matter of days. This eliminates a lot of occlusal adjustments during delivery. <u>Do not do this with your bridges</u> because you may not be able to count on this self-corrective action.

Crowns and bridges are your most profitable procedures. They are also great practice builders and self-rewarding techniques. On the other hand, they can be detrimental to your career, if performed injudiciously. I see plenty of expensive work being placed on periodontally involved teeth. At the same time, I see many ill-fitting margins causing deterioration and breakdown. Although patients do not always know what you are putting in their mouths, the next dentist will. Worse, their lawyer may know. Do everything possible to perform quality prosthetic work. Be your own worst critic.

While developing your rehabilitation skills with crowns and bridges, you should get in the habit of temporarily seating your work. Multiple unit bridges normally require patient acclimatization. If you seat the work permanently you are not going to be able to do any adjustments, other than occlusal. I like to seat most of my bridges temporarily. I **coat the abutments with Vaseline and then use Temp-Bond to seat the bridge**. I allow the patient to get used to the bridge for about a month and then if there are no problems (i.e. occlusion is good, shade is correct, sensitivity is non-apparent, and hygiene is appropriate) I will permanently seat it. I have had a few cases when the pulps flared up on me during the temporary stage. It was great to be able to remove the bridge, perform the root canal, and then seat the bridge without any holes and repairs. I have also had a few cases where the patient could not tolerate the porcelain. This happens in some patients. The porcelain is very hard and the opposing teeth do not adjust properly in occlusion - they hurt upon biting. It was nice to remake the work without having to cut everything off. Yes, new impressions were necessary!!!

If you have any doubts about your bridge, temporize it.

It is important for you to gain more crown and bridge knowledge.

Talk to your lab often and get their input about your work. Strive to improve constantly through feedback and education. My lab technician sends all of his family and friends to my office. This says a lot about my work.

SUCCESS CAN ONLY BE ACHIEVED WHEN ALL PARTS WORK TOGETHER

CHAPTER 32
EXTRACTIONS

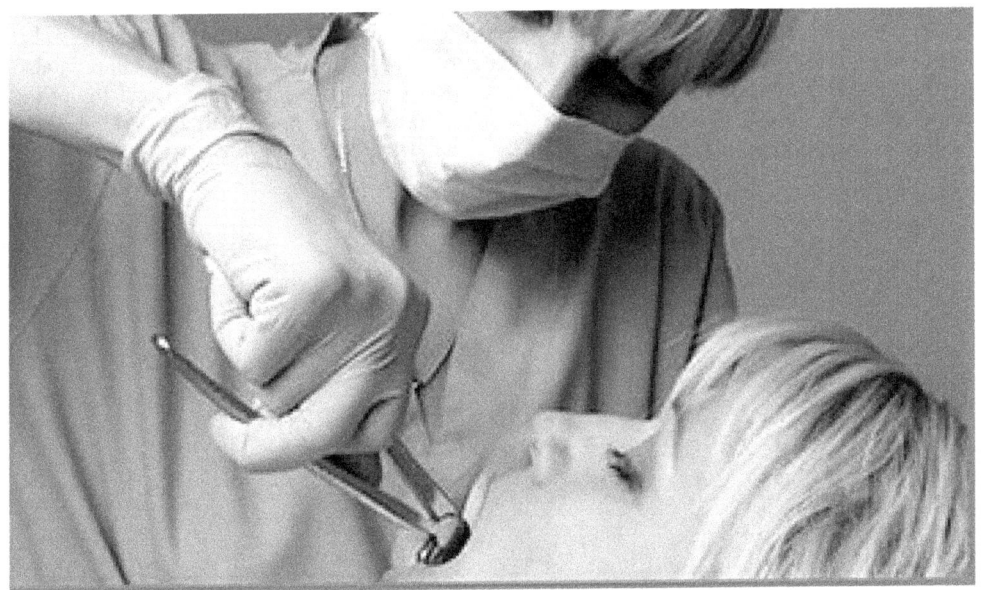

If you don't feel confident about extracting teeth, spend some time with your oral surgeon. Even the most benign looking extraction can turn into a surgical problem.

Knowledge of dental anatomy is critical to your ability to perform surgical extractions. Pre-op x-rays are your right hand. Know your limitations and don't get in over your head.

Stubborn teeth are usually calcified to the bone or have curved roots. For lower molars, hemisection is usually the easiest way of removing the roots. If Big Foot is sitting in my chair and he has a lower molar that looks as big as my toe, I automatically take a 557 surgical bur and split the tooth into two parts. I remove the distal root first and then slowly elevate the mesial roots towards the distal. If the roots do not budge, even after hemisection, I start removing bone all the way around the root, as though I was doing a deep crown preparation. It is not always necessary to lay a more than a partial flap, unless the roots keep chipping and breaking and your access is poor. Usually, even the most stubborn tooth will loosen up after you have sectioned it and removed mesial and distal bone.

Upper molars usually require hemisection of each root. Cut the tooth in three equal parts and elevate the roots one at a time. If you have to remove bone around the tooth, be careful not to damage adjacent teeth. It is easy to penetrate the sinus with a surgical bur, especially in the furcation area. Try to do most of your bone reduction on the facial aspect of the facial cusps and palatal aspect of the palatal cusp. Root tip picks are very helpful. Keep in mind the position of the maxillary artery and nerve. If you suspect sinus encroachment, flap and try to get complete socket closure by pulling the flap up and over the extraction site. If you cannot do so, get your patient to the surgeon's office right away! Don't forget to have the patient purchase some decongestants.

X-rays should be taken to help you evaluate your progress, as well as your post-op results. I also like to use Gel-Foam to pack all sockets following bone reduction. A figure eight suture is also advised. Antibiotic prescription is a must. Pain meds are obviously necessary. Don't forget the Prednisone For smokers, even if I performed a simple extraction, I will always prescribe antibiotics and Peridex.

BE BRAVE

RECYCLE

AVOID SARCASM

AMUSE, DON'T ABUSE

CONTROL TEMPER

SHOW RESPECT

BIG THOUGHTS

SMALL PLEASURES MAKE THE WORLD GO AROUND

CHAPTER 33
PERIO

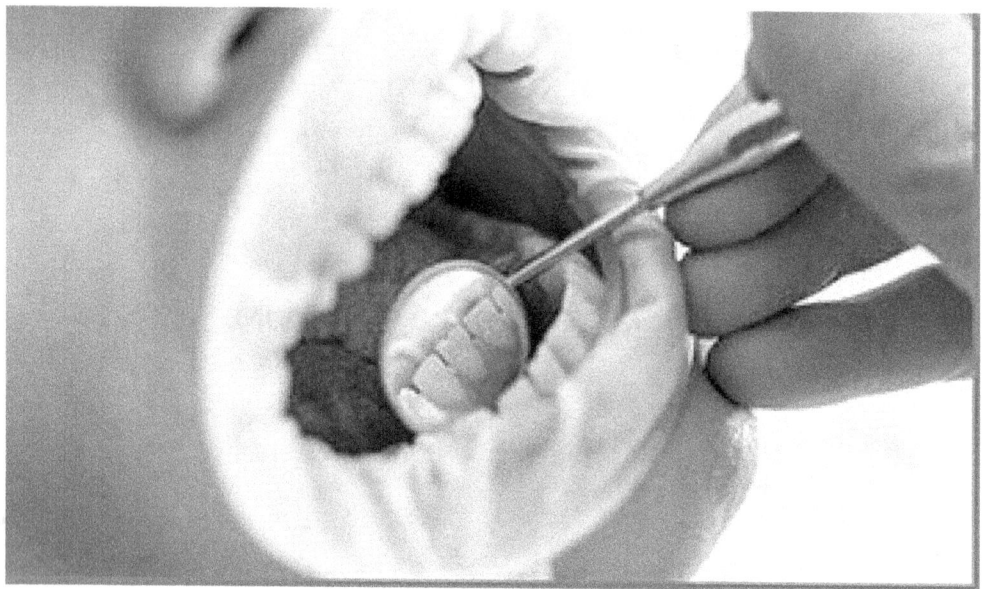

A house without foundation cannot be remodeled. A mouth without healthy gums cannot be restored.

You should be doing all of your scaling and root planing, without need for referral. Profound anesthesia is your key to success. I finish all of my perio cases in two visits. First visit, I numb from third molar to central incisor in the upper and lower quads on the same side. I regularly use palatal anesthesia and sometimes it is even necessary to use local infiltration around the lower teeth (besides the block). I use an ultrasonic handpiece along with plenty of Soft-Scale. Sharp scalers are critical to my efficiency. I will go through 4 or 5 scalers by the time I am done with 2 quadrants. **Glass-like root surfaces are the key to success.** You're not done until the scaler goes to the bone without any hang-ups or *rough encounters of the third kind*.

Don't be afraid to remove gum tissue during scaling. This is called curettage or gingivectomy in most insurance code books. Although most contracts do not allow for scaling, gingivectomy and curettage at the same visit (review chapter 17) I like to remove diseased tissue during scaling, because I do not feel that any patient deserves to go through periodontal treatment more than once. Some insurance contracts will allow for gingivectomy performed at the same visit with scaling, but they are rare. I do what is best for the patient and I ask them whether they want to wait that extra four weeks for healing as per their insurance contract, before performing any gum reduction. Most patients are delighted to pay the extra few hundred dollars and not have to go through more treatment. Sometimes, I don't even charge for the gingivectomy since I am chopping away at the calculus anyway.

The average gingivectomy performed during scaling takes only about an extra fifteen minutes. The bottom line is the need of the patient and their condition. If you think that a 9 mm. pocket can resolve with scaling and root planing then wait four weeks and see before you perform the gingivectomy. On the planet that I live on, any pocket above 7 mm. gets reduced during the scaling operation. Removing hyperplastic and infected gum tissue helps the healing and gives you great post-op results. Use your Laser.

I allow all of my perio cases at least twelve months of post-op care before I recommend any surgery. I like to see how the pockets resolve and how the patient hygiene progresses before I refer. It is rare that I refer a periodontal patient for flap surgery.

The main criteria for proceeding with further surgery are:

1. **Infrabony defects.**
2. **Unresolved pocket depths.**
3. **Patient's inability to clean the teeth and gums, due to pocketing.**

If your scaling and curettage/gingivectomy appointments were performed adequately, the need for further surgery is rare (except for advanced cases).

Be careful in evaluating furcation areas of your molars. Sometimes calculus build-up could mask and hide a beginning furcation problem. Spend time with your scaler when cleaning around the furcation areas.

A lot of your perio patients will benefit from bite splint therapy and equilibration. Recommend both treatments for optimal success!!!

Antibiotic therapy is very important during active treatment. My first choice is Amox 500 mg tid and I may also prescribe some Flagyl 250 bid for no more than 5 days. Peridex is very useful but make sure it is discontinued after active treatment, especially after the final polishing appointment. Doxycycline 100 mg bid is also a very good regimen and I like to use it for relapsed cases. Don't forget to have patient purchase ACT Fluoride and Sensodyne.

You should also get into the habit of brushing Fluoride on the newly exposed root surfaces in order to decrease cold sensitivity. Sometimes fluoride trays are very helpful if the patient is experiencing severe sensitivity. Make sure you don't kill the patient while taking the alginates. I recommend using warm water and slow set alginate to give you enough time to take the impression (remember: the warm water speeds up the alginate). Do these extra procedures for the comfort of your patients. Remember the marketing aspect of your practice.

None of your periodontal patients should finish treatment without purchasing an electric or sonic toothbrush. You may incorporate the fee for these items into the treatment and dispense them at the completion of care. Your post-op compliance and results will be much better. **Take the time**

to instruct your periodontal patients in proper home care. Dispenses toothbrushes, floss, floss-picks, and Proxabrushes. Most patients will find it easier to use floss-picks than floss. I see too many previous periodontal treatment patients coming from other offices where there was absolutely no hygiene education. This is a sin.

The most important aspect of successful periodontal treatment is patient compliance.

Spoon feed them, burp them, do whatever it takes to show these patients how to take care of their teeth. Why do you think they're in the mess that you are treating to begin with? Lack of education! Most of these patients do not even know how to hold the floss, least of all use a Proxa-Brush or other mechanical devices. Don't scold or laugh at their inability to coordinate their hand to brain function. Most of these patients need a lot of coaching and patience from you. This is especially important at recalls.

Again: never scold any of your patients when it comes to their poor hygiene.

And, remember: they're not your teeth. You're there to help them with their problem and guide them towards health. If they have no motivation to do so it is not your fault. Don't feel bad if you find that a lot of your periodontal treatment patients are not motivated enough to care for their oral condition. They're most likely not taking very good care of their health either. Document your findings, educate the patient, show concern, and go on to the next item on your agenda. But never scold, demean, chastise, or patronize your patients. Just document everything properly!

LUCK IS A RESULT OF HARD WORK

SAY 'THANK YOU' AND 'PLEASE'

NEVER GOSSIP

CHERISH OLD FRIENDS

SHOW DIGNITY

TREAT OTHERS THE WAY YOU WANT THEM TO TREAT YOU

FLOSS

LIVE MODESTLY

PLANT A TREE

CHAPTER 34
TMJ (TMD)

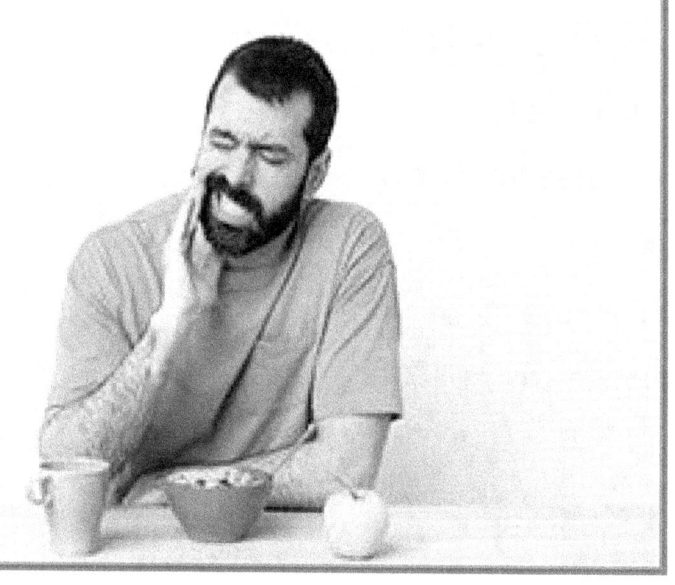

Abnormal masticatory systems are extremely common. Some may be acute, others subclinical. Regardless of clinical symptoms, TMD will have a tremendous affect on your dental work and your patient treatment protocol. It will also affect your patient's comfort and masticatory efficiency. **Dental treatment can aggravate existing TMJ conditions and can even unmask the dormant subclinical states, in some patients.** You must learn how to determine whether your patients have any form of TMD, in order to diagnose the serious risks accompanying dental treatment performed on undiagnosed TMD patients.

Recently, my associate had a young female patient who made an appointment for initial exam and possible fillings. Her oral condition was healthy, other than some mild abnormal enamel wear along with some tenderness in the masseter and medial pterygoid muscles. She stated previous episodes of joint pain accompanied by popping and clicking. The joints exhibited no abnormality at her appointment. He proceeded to finish four decayed occlusals with composites, upon her request. The same night this patient called complaining (actually screaming and crying) of severe headaches and orofacial pain. He immediately prescribed some Flexeril and Motrins. A day later she was still having pain. I saw her and realized that she was a chronic TMJ patient. I fitted her with a NTI. Her symptoms subsided. The patient was very thankful, despite the hardship she encountered. She respected my abililty to deal with her problem, as well as my expertise in TMJ treatment.

There are six basic etiologic factors for TMD:

1. Parafunctional habits (clenching, bruxing, lip biting, cheek biting, nail/pencil chewing, etc.).
2. Psychosocial and Psychological Factors (stress, depression, anxiety, social problems, etc.).
3. Systemic disorders (hormonal imbalances, arthritis, collagen disease, menopause, etc.).
4. Occlusal Disharmony
5. Trauma/Whiplash (accidents, extensive mouth opening, and prolonged mouth stretching).
6. Misaligned vertebrae (associated with any of the above or possible other systemic diseases).

In the past most TMJ experts agreed that Occlusal Disharmony was the cause of almost all TMD. Today, this belief has been discounted and disproved. TMD can and is caused by unbalanced occlusions, but you must have some of the other factors involved in order to overcome the body's compensatory mechanism. Many patients have unstable occlusions and never develop bruxism or joint popping. Many patients have very stable occlusions and have severe TMD problems. **From my 33+ years of experience: stress and Psychosocial factors are the leading causes of TMD problems.** Treating TMJ patients is not a very complicated modality, but you must have excellent people skills and lots of patience. Obviously, you need to spend a few hundred hours on continuing education on this topic.

TMJ therapy can be a great practice builder. It is not difficult to treat TMJ. Most of these patients normally require only a well-fitting bite splint and a little education. Some patients may require more extensive therapy, including physical, chiropractic, and possibly psychiatric treatment. In order to start treating a TMD patient you must learn how to conduct a thorough and unhurried TMJ examination. This includes physical examination, as well as patient screening and questionnaire evaluation.

Before you decide to proceed with your examination, know who you are treating.!!!

Don't open up the proverbial can of worms. Get to know the patient through an in-depth first exam visit. Don't begin to treat patients who may be out of your expertise. Evaluate the TMJ questionnaire carefully and sit down and talk with the patient. There are many TMD patients who you should not treat because they will make you lose sleep at night. If you don't feel comfortable treating the patient, REFER! If you decide to proceed, then complete your analysis and keep the following in mind:

1. What is the chief complaint?
2. When did the pain start, what time of day does it occur, and how often does it occur?
3. How intense is the pain and where is the pain?
4. What factors intensify or cause the pain?
5. Does anything alleviate the pain?
6. What parafunctional habits does this patient have?
7. What is this patient's occupation?
8. How is the health of this patient?
9. What previous injuries did patient suffer?
10. Are there noticeable noises around the TMJ?

11. Any episodes of locked jaw?
12. What about headaches (where, when, severity, frequency)?

TMJ treatment begins with a complete exam. The exam must be coordinated with the separate patient questionnaire, which focuses on the subjective problems associated with TMJ. This involves palpating the muscles of mastication for tenderness/pain, evaluating the joint for abnormalities, assessing the maximum opening, observing the range of mandibular movement, examining the dentition (as described in the first part of this book), and assessing the neck musculature. A lot of TMJ patients exhibit tenderness in the medial pterygoids and lateral pterygoids. This is due to their anterior bruxism habit. Once the musculature has been evaluated, take a stethoscope and listen to the opening and closing sounds of the joint itself. Crepitation and " creaking" sounds may indicate pathology. If there is no capsular involvement your main course of treatment will be to relax the musculature and "break" their habit. This is the standard of care for most of these patients.

Also pay attention to the neck and shoulder muscles. Tight trapezius and occipital muscles cause tension and bruxism. The cervical plexus of nerves can become very irritated in these patients and you will get secondary irritation of the trigeminal nerve because the cervical nerves meet the trigeminal nerve at the subnucleus caudalis before entering the brain. There is a lot of correlation between the neck/shoulder area and the muscles of mastication.

Once you are done assessing the motor function and your head/neck examination is completed, take another look at the occlusion. What is the maximum opening? What about crossbites and open bites? Are there wear facets and balancing interferences? Look at the anterior teeth a little closer and see how much uneven wear they exhibit.

Once your TMJ assessment is completed you have to begin your counseling and patient education session. **You cannot have any success treating TMJ unless you educate your patient and get their full cooperation and understanding.** I educate all of my patients in regard to how their muscles work, how nerve impulses stimulate the nerves, and how the teeth can and be affected by the muscles. I also emphasize how stress and demands of daily life can take their toll on the TMJ. The affected muscles are not only the oro-facial ones but also the neck and back musculature. The patient must comprehend this and they must also be educated in respect to caffeine and sugar consumption.

Although the above paragraphs paint a simplistic view of TMJ, you will find that most of your TMJ patients fall into the category of people that I call *strung-out*. The majority of my TMD patients are females who work two jobs and have a lot of stress in their lives. If you think that you can treat these patients with a bite appliance you are dreaming. You must eliminate many causative factors before you can have any treatment success. **Get to know your patient**. You will find that your typical TMJ patient consumes large amounts of stimulants and has a very hectic lifestyle. You must counsel these patients and become a pseudo-therapist. I am not telling you to go out and get a psychology degree, but you need above average people skills and bed-side manners in order to be able to develop a great rapport with these patients. You must also develop some coaching skills to help these patients realize their condition.

TMJ patients usually have other health problems. The most common is neck and back pain. Tight trapezius muscles along with back pain is almost always noticed. TMJ involves more than just the muscles of mastication. As a simple approach, recommend the following to your patient:

1. Complete Physical by Physician to rule out any other health problems, especially glandular and psychological.
2. Assessment by Physical Therapist. Let the therapist show the patient how to improve spinal posture, neck posture, and give the patient a home-based exercise program. Visit your physical therapist often and learn how they assess patients. Find a therapist who stresses exercise programs, strengthening, and postural rehabilitation. Posture is key!!! Many therapists are not skilled in treating TMJ, but it does not take an Einstein to learn how to massage the muscles of mastication and get them to relax. Teach a capable therapist how to perform stretch and massage therapy. Usually the therapist will find many other muscular problems besides the TMJ problem. Let them work on all of the problems, because the TMJ is usually very minor.
3. Review sleeping posture. The optimal sleeping position is with very minimal neck support and on your back. Most TMJ patients sleep on their side and their stomach, usually with their necks propped up by many pillows. Get them to throw out their pillows. A rolled up towel is the best neck support. Get your patient to sleep on their back!!! If they sleep on a waterbed tell them to toss it out of the window.
4. Avoid caffeine and sugar!!!
5. No TV at least 2 hours before bed-time.
6. Purchase back support orthotic pillows and wear while driving and while seated. If your patient sits in a chair at work, get them to review their sitting posture and purchase a chair recommended by their physical therapist.
7. Visit a chiropractor at least once a week. Get to know the chiropractor! If this professional does not believe in "specific" adjustments find another one. The optimal chiropractic care includes adjustments of specific vertebrae in order to get long-term benefits. There are very few chiropractors that can perform a complete spinal exam and adjust appropriately.
8. Eliminate stressful events, one at a time.
9. Lips together, teeth apart, no apples.
10. If work involves computer screens, purchase an antiglare cover.
11. Vitamins, nutrition, and exercise.
12. Vacation.
13. "Counseling," if the patient feels that they need it, or if they request it. Be careful about making this recommendation. You could end up losing the patient. Be tactful. Get to know family members who may be more open to making this suggestion to the patient. Obviously some TMJ patients are already suffering from psychiatric problems. I will never refer a patient for psychiatric treatment or counseling. Most of these patients already know their problem and usually are under treatment to begin with. Psychiatric evaluation is out of the scope of dental treatment, in my opinion. Let the patient's physician handle it. The medical doctor can make the appropriate referral to the psychologist, psychiatrist, or neurologist.

Obviously you want to make sure that these patients have optimal dental health because that is usually the reason that they came to your office to begin with. If these patients require restorative work and their TMJ problems are acute, DON'T DO IT!!! Not until you can calm down the TMJ problem and get them more comfortable. Even an occlusal amalgam can become a major deal. Don't open up the worm can. JUST DON'T DO IT!

All TMJ patients require bite splint therapy. Over 38% of the nerve impulses that reach other parts of the body travel near the TMJ. An inflamed or damaged TMJ will directly affect many other bodily functions, and vice versa. You must attempt to relieve pressure in and around the joint. The muscles must be relaxed and blood flow must be improved. A properly fitted splint can help relax the oral musculature and provide relief to the teeth. Over 80% of TMD patients will benefit from bite splint therapy, if performed properly. An improperly fitted splint can have devastating effects and worsen the condition. For simple cases of bruxism make an upper Astron bite splint with occlusion only for anteriors and NO contact on posterior teeth.

For complex cases that involve joint problems refer out or learn more about complex TMJ treatment.

Do NOT engage in occlusal equilibrations or fixing patient's bites unless you fully understand TMJ.

COMPLIMENT TWO PEOPLE EACH DAY

BE THANKFUL FOR WHAT YOU HAVE

PAY FOR QUALITY

ENJOY QUALITY

PRAISE QUALITY

BECOME A LEADER

THINK POSITIVE

WORDS HAVE POWER; USE THEM POSITIVELY

ENJOY THE FRUITS OF YOUR LABORS

LIFE IS SHORT; REALLY, IT IS!

CHAPTER 35
OCCLUSION

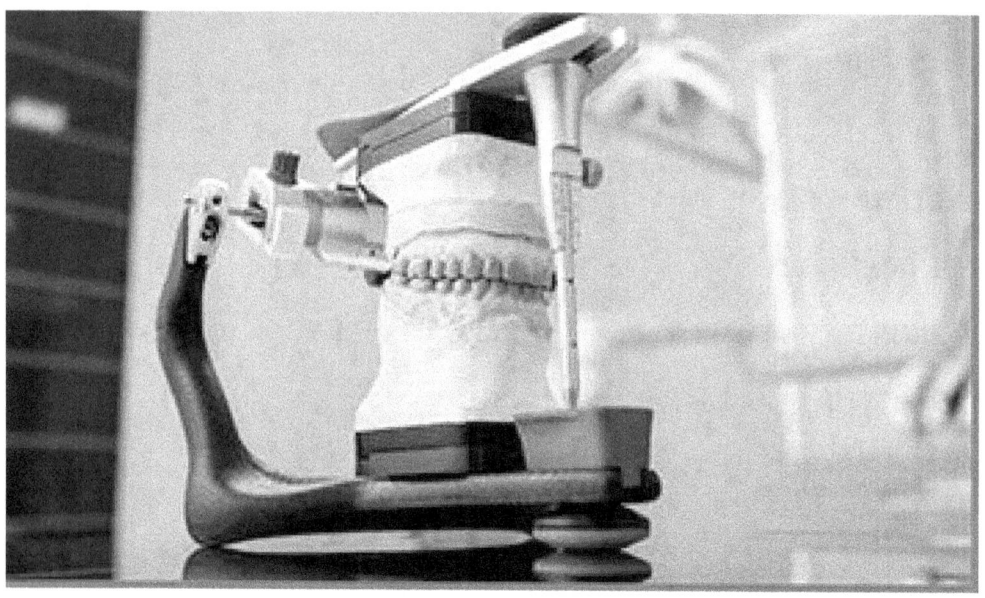

Modern dentistry offers a variety of possible ways to improve appearance and mastication. These possibilities have been improved through advancements in bonding agents and cosmetic materials. Before covering any other topics of clinical dentistry I would like to make you aware of the effects of anterior guidance and occlusal harmony.

Many patients want to have longer, fuller smiles. Desirable lengths vary according to personal desires. Average length for upper centrals is about 11 to 12 mm., while the laterals are about 9.5 to 10.5 mm. The cuspids are in the ballpark of about 11 to 12 mm. Patients with worn dentitions present with teeth much smaller in length than these averages. These patients may exhibit some form of TMJ problems such as bruxism or clenching. Some may be acute, others subclinical. In order to restore these patients you must assess the TMJ and occlusal scheme carefully. Adequately mounted study models are essential in planning these cases, as well as all of the rest of your complex restorative work. Face-bow transfer and CR bites are critical because you will be rebuilding these patients' jaw movements. Cuspid guidance must be your goal whenever possible. Anterior guidance must be evaluated and position/movement of the joints/jaw must be ascertained. Wax-ups are necessary to see how you can obtain *ideal guidance*. If cuspid guidance is not possible then treatment plan group function. As a general rule: Never place more than 2 crown and bridge units without assessing anterior guidance and jaw movements.

Other helpful ideas:

1. Restore posterior teeth only after you have finished the anterior segments and you have established anterior guidance. Temporize the posteriors while finishing the anteriors.
2. Consult with your lab.
3. Make friends with your prosthodontist.
4. Take time to see the forest from the trees. There is way too much single tooth dentistry done in this country. Learn to see the whole mouth and how it works as a unit and not as separate, single teeth.
5. Contact my office if you are in need of further prostho training.

SAVE 15% OF YOUR INCOME

RUN YOUR OWN LIFE, NOT THE LIFE OF OTHERS

BE PREPARED

BE ORGANIZED

CARRY PEN AND PAPER WITH YOU

CARRY CALENDAR WITH YOU

BE COMFORTABLE ASKING FOR HELP

LAUGH, SMILE, JOKE

LOOK IN THE MIRROR

CHAPTER 36
DENTURES/PARTIALS

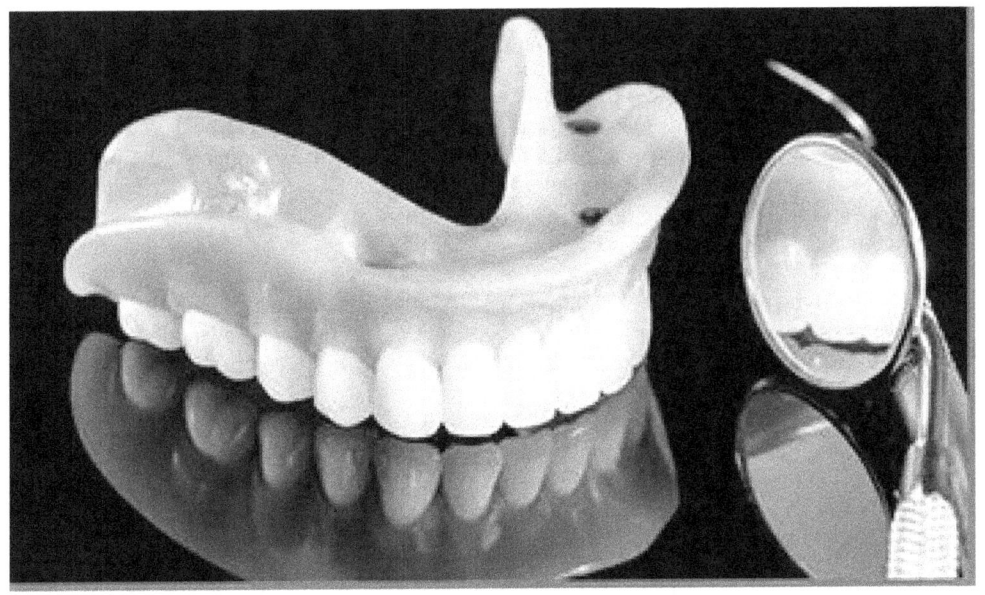

The most profitable and easiest procedures are partials and dentures. A couple of impressions and you're half done. The rest is up to your lab...WRONG!!!

Treatment plan your cases, especially partials. Don't fabricate partials without finishing your restorative and oral rehabilitation treatment. Think in terms of 5 years. Your patient should not develop any problems in their mouth for at least 5 years. Questionable teeth should be extracted and all restorative should be finished.

Design your partials. Don't let your lab plan your cases. You know what's best for your patient, not your lab.

Impression taking is the most important part of making good fitting partials and dentures. Again, remember: the entire mouth must be clean before you impress!!!

You must have a cooperative patient in order to get a good impression. **If you have a "gagger" then have them swallow some salt and spray a little anesthetic in their throat.** The salt is very helpful! For my denture impressions I use the Accu-Dent impression kit. These impressions are basically glorified alginates. They're easy on the patient and you're done in 10 minutes. I haven't border molded since senior year in school. The kit and instructions are self-explanatory. Your only obstacle is to choose the right tray. Always use the largest trays possible.

During impression taking, push the trays as far as possible into the roof of the mouth and as low as possible on the lower. Pull the cheeks tightly over the tray and you should have a perfect impression. These impressions are basically a functional impression because you are capturing the entire arch at one time. These impressions usually give you even more detail and extension than you want, but your lab can always reduce this later. Undercuts are more evident with this impression technique because you are using resilient alginate.

Once you get a great impressions, the rest of your case depends on establishing vertical dimension. Take your time! Have the patient enunciate your basic words: "Mississippi," "59," "55," "69," "semi-sweet," etc. Once you can get the patient in rest vertical you can easily measure your centric occlusion. I use two tongue blades for my measurements. The first, I hold vertical, beginning with light pressure under the nose (pick a stable spot and duplicate it). The second, I use horizontally (under the chin) to record the actual vertical dimension. I keep the patient talking as I record the rest vertical with a pencil line where my horizontal blade meets the vertical blade. I try to maintain the horizontal blade very steady as the patient talks. This can best be accomplished by using one finger mid-way between the chin and neck. Don't allow this blade to sway. Once I mark my rest vertical dimension, I subtract 2 mm. and draw another line on the blade with an arrow pointing upwards. This reminds me where my centric occlusion is when I put the wax bite in the mouth.

Placing wax bite rims in the patient's mouth is sometimes a difficult task. It is not easy to get an edentulous patient to duplicate their jaw movement correctly, especially when the large wax rims are tugging and ballooning their mouths. The patient's proprioception is often affected. I try to fabricate the lightest and smallest bite trays possible. After I put them in the mouth I check to see where my vertical dimension is. Often, I have to trim the thickness of one or both of the wax rims. When I have achieved the appropriate dimension, I practice with the patient to help them give me a proper recording. Having the patient stick their tongue to the roof of their mouth while opening and closing is usually the best way to help them regulate their opening and closing movement. Once I feel that the patient can easily duplicate the movement, I add yellow bite wax to the upper rim and notch the lower rim. I place the lower in the mouth, then the upper, and slowly guide the patient into centric relation. It may be necessary to use some Fixodent to make the rims retentive.

You do not want to hold the trays for the patient with your fingers. This will lead to false movements of the mandible. I like to take the bite at least two or three times in order to verify the correctness. If you have a severely atrophic mandible and/or maxilla you should have the assistant hold the uppers at the premolar region, while you hold the lower steady and guide the patient into biting.

I can't emphasize how important it is to have nice fitting and comfortable bite wax rims. **The whole case will depend on your bite.** There may be some cases that you will have to reset despite your best efforts. The set-up comes back from the lab and the occlusion is way off. The best way to retake a bite is to **remove the lower molars**, add some yellow wax and have the patient bite down without any assistance. If you leave the molars they may throw the bite off since they contact first, thereby throwing off the patient's proprioception.

Be your own worst critic when evaluating the set-up. The first criteria you should assess is the placement of the lower occlusal scheme. **Remember the retromolar pad.** All of your impressions (for partials and dentures) should show this anatomical landmark. **All lower teeth should be set 1 or 2 mm. below a horizontal plane that starts at the level of the retromolar pad.** If your lab has followed this basic rule of set-up the remaining aspect of your esthetics relies upon your vertical dimension and shape/size of your teeth.

Some patients may request more or less of a smile line. Do whatever possible to achieve patient requests, but keep in mind the basics of functionality and fit. Have the patient go through all speech patterns. **If you hear too many "s" sounds your vertical may be too closed - you need to close the articulator down a little and provide more freeway space.** Check to make sure that the teeth are not set too far to the lingual or possibly the lowers may be too far above the occlusal plane (check that retromolar pad landmark).

The lower lip should just touch the uppers when the patient pronounces "55." Use this word to help you assess the smile line. Also check the patient's cheek and lip for proper support. Some patients may require more support, others may feel uncomfortable with extra bulkiness. You should discuss this during the bite appointment, before you have the lab do the set-up. Never hurry your denture patients, especially during the try-in appointment. Make sure you allow them to look in the mirror, walk around, get family member input, and study their new mouth. Make all changes that the patient requests, and do not hurry. Once the patient is satisfied with the set-up have them sign the chart to indicate their approval.

<u>Make sure that all fees have been collected!!!</u>

Denture patients can become difficult patrons at your office. Do everything possible to make the dentures comfortable during delivery. Remove all undercuts and check extensions to make sure that they are not too long. A lot of dentures require long extensions only on the lingual borders of the lowers and the pterygoid hamular process of the uppers. The other borders should be trimmed to where the cheek attaches to the attached gingiva. You don't want your cheeks pulling on the dentures.

If the upper is loose, check the hamular extension and the posterior seal. One of these is usually inadequate. If the lower is unretentive see if you have made the lingual flange long enough to get under the tongue and grab unto the lingual part of the mandible. <u>Trim the buccal extensions of your lower plate so that the cheeks don't push up on the denture!!!</u>

Don't forget to adjust the occlusion!!! Even the best fitting dentures will cause problems if the occlusion is not correct.

Partial dentures may require more planning and preliminary work. Make sure you have stable teeth and a good design. A excellent alginate is critical!!! Remember to double check your occlusion for hypererupted teeth. The success of your partials depends on your occlusion. Attempt to have an even occlusal plane whenever possible...you'll see less broken teeth and clasps in the future.

I rarely use rest seats for my partials. They load the tooth too much and sometimes interfere with seating. Tight clasps, indirect retention, and perfectly fitted bases are the keys to patient comfort. I always use butt-gum designs for anterior teeth on partials to help me achieve great esthetics. Take time to refine your set-up.

Make your partials look invisible and watch your referrals come out of the woodwork.

Sometimes it is necessary to use metal-backed porcelain facings for some partials on patients with strong bites and collapsed occlusions. Treatment plan these for success, otherwise your plastic teeth will keep breaking. For tight occlusions it is O.K. to leave occlusal bites on metal extensions. You don't always have to put a tooth into place, especially in the posterior. Metal occlusal stops, along with metal-backed porcelain teeth, will prolong the life of your partials and prevent follow-up repairs.

Don't forget to have your lab make you a customized shade guide for your gum color. Custom gum-shade matching is critical to the final esthetics. White people don't always have pink gums and black people don't always have brown gums. **Pay attention to gum color. Get your patient's input.**

The last and most important thing: pay your lab a visit, when necessary. I stop by my lab at least once every two weeks, or more often if I have a difficult case. It is important to communicate with your lab. Don't expect your lab person to figure out your cases for you.

And I have a strict policy for all denture patients: *Pay before you play.* If you allow your denture patients to make payments on their dentures, or if you allow them to leave over half of their payment responsibility for their last appointment, you may encounter some patients who just can't find anything right with their denture. Don't set up payment plans for any denture patients.

Denture relines are also great practice builders. You don't always have to send the case to the laboratory. There are many fine materials that allow you to do a cold-cure reline intraorally. For soft liners I use PermaSoft. For hard liners I have used Hygenic and Tokuso.

Make sure you mix the hard liners to a very thin consistency otherwise you will be rebasing dentures and making them feel like a ton of bricks in the patient's mouth. Another helpful hint is to make three *escape holes* in your dentures. Make them at least 5 mm. in diameter. For uppers I cut two holes in the distal most extension of the ridges and at the incisive papilla. For lowers, anywhere is OK, just space them apart. These holes provide relief vents for the reline material to flow through and will give you much better relines as the tissues will not be so compressed because the reline material will flow with ease. Place these holes even if you are taking a rubber base impression and sending the case to the lab. Give the impression material a chance to flow without resistance and you will get an excellent reline.

Also be certain that you put a lot of pressure on the prosthesis in order to push it tightly on the arch. When you do lab relines use the old Permlastic Light Body Rubber Base technique for the impression. It is still the best material for this procedure. Double check your extensions and coverages. If you need to extend the hamular area or the lower retromolar pad you can use some impression compound sticks (the ones you made friend with in dental school border molding) and border mold the denture to cover these areas better. Re-verify your occlusion and rest vertical dimensions.

CHAPTER 37
ESTHETICS

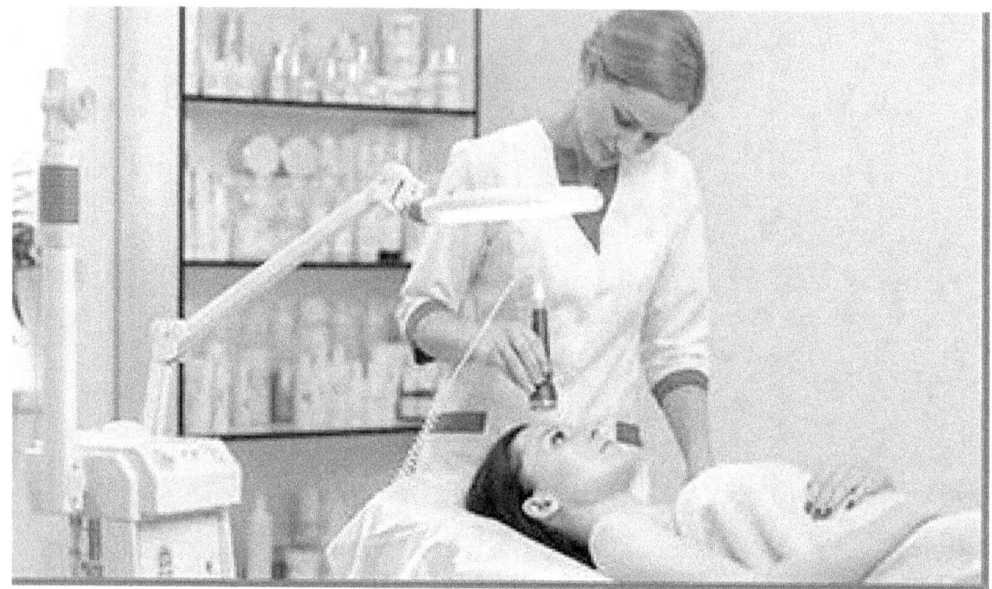

The practitioner who does not become proficient at performing cosmetic dentistry will be left in the dust. Over half of my practice is now cosmetic dentistry. Although I strongly urge practitioners to be careful about jumping into cosmetic dental work, I believe that you have to develop your skills in this area. After you have done a few thousand amalgams, root canals, PFM crowns, gold inlays/onlays, you can start to look at this area of dentistry. However, until you have mastered the art of the bread and butter stuff you should not begin doing cosmetic dentistry. Cosmetic dental care involves a lot of skill, patience, and cost. It also involves proper treatment planning and appropriate case selection. Failures will kill your overhead.

There are a lot of speakers and experts trying to preach the benefits of cosmetic dentistry. Take a lot of these sermons with a glass of bitter wine because when you go back to your office you will wake up to reality and see that there are not too many patients waiting to put a few thousand dollars of porcelain veneers in their mouths. You must do a lot of education to be able to perform cosmetic dentistry. Even then, you will not find a lot of patients opting for these treatment options.

When I have a patient with un-perceived cosmetic needs I normally take a few minutes to do an intra-oral mock-up bonding. This is very simple. Place some composite on the dry teeth in question without etching, bonding, or curing. All you need is a wet-gloved-finger or brush. This can show the patient what they can possibly look like with esthetic bonding or porcelain work. It is also helpful to take a photo of this mock-up and send it home with the patient. For better results you can also have your local lab do computer images for you. This is the best marketing and educational tool that you can use to start selling cosmetic dental work.

Before you begin any cosmetic procedures take a close look at the patient's overall dental status, especially occlusion and possible parafunctional habits. Interferences and uneven occlusal schemes will ruin your cosmetic work! Review Dr. Christensen's Occlusal Equilibration Tapes and read Dr. Dawson's books. Get in the habit of doing careful occlusal analysis.

Do not perform extensive cosmetic work in an unbalanced mouth.

Never perform cosmetic dentistry in a mouth with poor hygiene!!!

My office is full of before and after books, along with cosmetic posters and brochures. Your patients will love to look through some of these photo albums and literature. Get them talking about esthetic dental procedures. Purchase some professionally produced albums and start to develop your own photo albums!

I practically give away bleaching kits. Almost all patients that bleach their teeth return for more expensive work or refer other patients in need of these services. It is my best advertising. It is also my foundation for starting cosmetic work. All veneer cases undergo preop bleaching.

At our office we have the GLO product available for purchase. If the patient requests deeper whitening products then we fabricate lab made trays or use the KOR system

We do NOT offer amalgams for posterior restorative. Composites make great restorations and the only difficulty is the contact area. To compensate for light contacts, wedge the teeth as tight as possible and use very thin metal matrix bands. Burnish the matrix bands against the neighboring tooth and loosen the fit of the band without losing cervical adaptation. Use the ball burnisher to push the matrix against the adjacent tooth during filling. Cure as you hold the ball burnisher and you'll have a great contact. Review chapter 28.

Never perform cosmetic dentistry in a mouth with poor hygiene. It will come back to haunt you. All of your cosmetic patients should be on a regular program of fluoride rinses and six month recalls. Pick your patients wisely. Cosmetic work will fail in a mouth that is not being taken care of.

With today's contact thin porcelain options veneers are easy to complete and highly profitable, especially if done in multiple units. Composites can also be used to accomplish amazing results.

First, and foremost, **never be afraid to reduce enamel** especially on cases where the patient does not want bulky teeth. Even for thin veneers you must create a slight margin up to the cervical and into the contact area and hide your finish lines in these areas for excellent results.

Obviously your cosmetic work will depend on selecting the right shade. Are your eyes good enough to match the appearance of natural teeth? Young women see these variations the best. As you age things look more yellow and brown. If you drink coffee it may affect your perception, as well. To understand colors, review some of your dental school basics.

HUE: the old ROYGBIV
CHROMA: saturation (kind of like water coloring - how red can it get?)
VALUE: brightness (black being low brightness and white being high brightness)

Value is the most important!!! Arrange your shade guides this way, in decreasing VALUE:

B1 A1 B2 D2 A2 C1 C2 D4 A3 D3 B3 A3.5 B4 C3 A4 C4

Use color corrected light in your operatories (day-light bulbs) to give you more precise measurements. It is also helpful to stare at blue colors for five seconds to rest your eyes. Not longer than 5 seconds!

When shaping your teeth, first start out by evaluating the line angles. This is where the facial meets the interproximal. To make tooth <u>wider</u> flatten the facial and add composite to the line angles to bulk them up a little. To make the tooth look <u>narrower</u> round out the facial and decrease the bulk at the line angles. To make the tooth look <u>longer</u> bulk up the cervical and flatten the incisal half. To make the tooth look <u>shorter</u>, bulk up the incisal half and flatten the cervical part.

The embrasures are also very important. The incisal and cervical meeting of adjacent teeth will affect the overall appearance of the smile. Each tooth has 4 embrasures on the buccal and 4 on the lingual. Attempt to make these even and uniform on all of the anteriors.

<u>Before you start to finish your esthetic restorations get up out of the chair, sit the patient up, and take a close look at your work from the **front of the patient**. Your chair-side position can give you a slanted view and you could end up obliquing your work. Get the patient out of the chair and take a look at them while standing up. Take a pencil and draw any lines or marks to help you achieve proper contour and line angles.</u>

Last, but not least, POLISH all of your composites. Using ample water irrigation learn to polish your composites to the point where they look glass-like. Start <u>gross</u> reduction with fine diamonds, go to your 12-fluted carbides or sand disks, then finish up with Enhance cups and disks and gloss-paste. Remember to keep the tooth cool!

<u>For more advanced cases, especially when doing porcelain veneers, here are some extra suggestions.</u>

- Tomorrow I want you to call your lab and make an appointment to spend some time with the technicians. Look at model preps and get some insight from these people. You will be amazed at what they can teach you!!!

- The smile line is a critical element. It is formed by the <u>incisal edges</u> and it should follow the lip in a rounded fashion from midline backwards. The posteriors should not look like they're going to fall into the mandible as they go back. Look at the lips!!!

- The buccal corridor is the space between the maxillary posterior teeth and the inner cheek. If this space is too big you will see a dark tunnel when you smile. You esthetics should include bulking up of the facials, if necessary. Treatment plan veneers on your bicuspids for optimal results.

- The size and proportion of your teeth is always the most important aspect of preparing your cosmetic work. As a general rule your teeth should be proportionate to each other when viewed two dimensionally (i.e. in a photograph or on this piece of paper). Your centrals should be 1.6 times larger than your laterals, and your cuspids should look .6 times the size of your laterals. In other words if you have a lateral that is 7 mm. then your central should be 11.2 mm. (7 times 1.6) while your cuspid should appear at 4.2 mm. (7 times .6). This is obviously not their real size, but what they look like from the front in a two dimensional perspective.

- Your teeth must also be proportionate to themselves. If you divide the width of the tooth by the length you should achieve a Width to Length Ratio of approximately 75- 80%. If this percentage is higher than 80% you must decrease the width and increase the length. If you percentage is lower than 75% than you must increase the width and decrease the length. Measure the width and length of each tooth individually!!!

- How is the midline? Can you correct it?

- What about the axial inclination? Teeth should have a slight backward inclination from mesial to distal when observing them from the front. Draw a vertical line through the middle of each tooth. If these lines do not appear parallel and slightly leaning backwards at the cervicals, on each side, than you have to plan for readjustment.

- Finally, check the gingival contour. Make sure to prepare for gum shaping if the gingival roll is not aligned properly. You must achieve an even height of gingiva if you want your restorations to look proportionate. An electrosurgery unit or laser is a must.

- When you are ready to start doing porcelain work, visit your lab. See what they recommend and learn to work with the systems that they prefer using. Emax is the most popular esthetic porcelain at the time of the release of this book.

One more bit of advice: PFM crowns are beautiful restorations if you know how to do a nice deep chamfer margin on the buccals and hide the finish line about 1 mm. into the gum. They can actually provide better opaquing of cervical areas for discolored teeth especially when you have metal posts and cores. Obsidian crowns made by Glidewell are awesome restorations.

CHAPTER 38
ALL-PORCELAIN CROWNS AND VENEERS

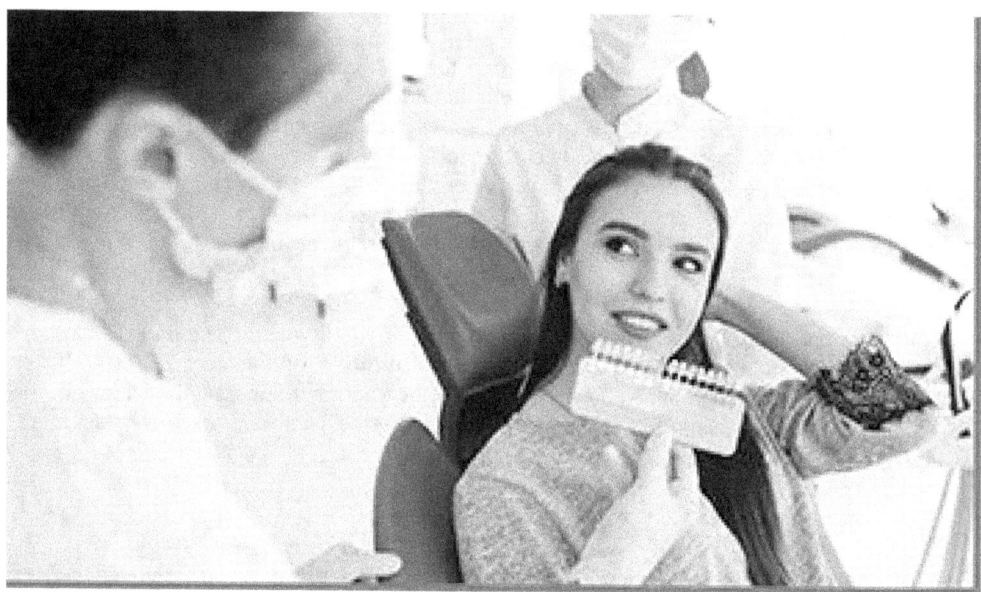

If you are planning on becoming a "cosmetic" dentist I suggest that you take at least 10 hands-on continuing education courses before you begin any porcelain work. Check with your local commercial laboratory and ask for their advice. However, be careful before you give anyone thousands of dollars to teach you something that you may not be able to provide. Most large labs, such as Glidewell, also have continuing education seminars on this topic. Call your local lab, first. Spend a few days with the quality control manager. Check out AGD listings, as well. This is a fast changing area in dentistry. Keep abreast of developments because they happen fast. Esthetic dentistry is tedious, time consuming work that requires talent and skill. It can be very profitable if it is performed properly, but it can also be unprofitable if it is done hurriedly and non-attentively.

There are not going to be a lot of patients coming to your office begging for your cosmetic services. Few patients can afford veneers and porcelain restorations that are not covered by insurance contracts. This is one of the reasons that you should concentrate on developing your bread and butter skills before you decide to improve your cosmetic expertise. You are not going to make a living trying to perform multiple veneers on your middle class patients. Nevertheless, you should learn how to treatment plan and complete cosmetic cases to the best of your ability.

If you want to provide a superior looking restoration for an anterior tooth **think Emax or Zirconia Esthetic.** I use Emax for all single unit anterior procedures when the tooth is not grossly discolored, non-root canaled, and there is no evidence of bruxism or unusual occlusal wear. If the tooth has a discolored core I usually stay with the PFM crown (Obsidian). If the patient is a bruxer I use the Zirconia Esthetic.

Before you begin to prepare a tooth for porcelain coverage you must have complete gingival health and stable occlusion. Bleeding gums and perio pocketing will come back to haunt you. Reduce all gum depths to under 3 mm before you begin porcelain work, especially in the anterior region.

Unbalanced occlusions can fracture any porcelain crown! Always use Zirconia if the occlusion is not stable and/or the patient exhibits signs of abnormal wear secondary to bruxism or parafunctional habits. Get into thinking about what happens to your work after the patient walks out of the door. Think about occlusal contacts, function, and bad habits (i.e. pencil chewing, pipe smoking, etc.).

Mount your study models and discuss the case with your lab technician!
Fabricate "clearance" vacuum shells and practice the preps on the working models.

Another preliminary analysis you must make is the contour of your gums - the gingival roll. Does the shape and contour of the gingival area flow smoothly and evenly? Does your patient desire to have longer looking teeth? Are there any dehiscence problems or erosion areas? **The free gingival margin contour, shape, and roll will directly affect the final appearance of your work.** You can make teeth longer by removing gingiva. You can create an even flow by making sure that the position of the gingival margin is at the same level from premolars to premolars. The laser is your best friend for correcting the shape, contour and position of your free gingival margin. If you feel that contouring the gums will give the patient a fuller smile and/or correct the shape of the gums in the quadrant, treatment plan this step to allow for healing - before you begin the preparations. You must wait at least 2 weeks for adequate healing. Almost all of my big veneer cases (4 or more units) normally receive some sort of gingival contouring surgery.

Another criteria for placing all-porcelain crowns is your ability to match the shade of adjacent teeth. This is very difficult to do when you have other porcelain or PFM crowns in the same area. An all-porcelain crown will be very hard to match next to a PFM crown. If the patient has a PFM crown on #8 and you're thinking of putting an all-porcelain crown on #9 get ready to use color modifiers, try-in pastes, and gypsy powders before choosing the final cement color. Better yet, treatment plan re-make of the PFM for optimal esthetics.

The preparation for any crown is basically the same. The only difference is when you have to hide root discoloration...remove more tooth structure and provide the lab technician with more "room" to opaque the area. A 2.0 mm. shoulder or chamfer type shoulder is often necessary for such teeth.

Measure the width of your diamonds to give you an idea how to use them as "tracers." Visit your lab and ask them to show you study models of ideal preparations. Absorb these into your cerebellum. Practice some preps on extracted teeth.

When doing porcelain veneers, the criteria for cementation are the same. The main difference is the preparation. Veneer preparations require adequate reduction, but not as much as a full porcelain crown. You always want to leave the enamel contact intact. You should not be afraid to remove tooth structure when doing porcelain veneers, but you should keep the preparation in enamel and not in dentin. Don't tell your patients that veneers require very little to no tooth removal. A beautiful veneer for stained teeth requires almost 1 mm. of reduction, especially for any gray shades.

Pay careful attention your facial contours and margins during veneer preparation. You may need to reduce your facial margin at least .75mm to not make the teeth bulkier. You should always prep the margin right up to the gingival margin and make sure that your gingiva is healthy.

I DO NOT like to "wrap" the incisal edges with porcelain if at all possible. The main reason for this is due to the anterior protrusive contact of the lowers against this margin. Over a five year period it will create a crater between the porcelain and the enamel. Sometimes you may have to wrap into the lingual for better esthetics, but try to finish your margin as far incisally as possible.

Think of your preparation as Lee Nails. Veneers are the dental equivalent of fake nails.

You should visit you lab and study porcelain preparations on the study models that they have. When you go to your next state association dental meeting spend time studying all of the different study models that the labs have on display. There are many preparations for all of the different variety of crowns that labs in your area can perform. This is the best way to visualize the required preparations for optimal esthetics.

Cementing PFM or porcelain crowns is now all the same. Revisit Chapter 28.
For veneers, a different approach is used.

1. Internal aspects of the crown must be etched with HF acid, not phosphoric, in order to achieve a good bonding surface.
2. Use silane coupling agent to improve the chemical bond of the cement to the porcelain
3. Etch, prime/bond the enamel and/or dentin. Remember to seal the dentin and enamel.
4. Fill the crown completely with cement (nexxus) and let it extrude upon seating. Wave your curing light over the area to start slight polymerization
5. Clean as much cement as possible after curing,
6. Allow the cement to start hardening for 2 minutes and then cure for at least 2 minutes from facial and lingual (use 2 lights).
7. Remove excess cement with a knife or thin, flame-shaped finishing burs or fine diamonds.
8. Double check all areas of the crown for left-over cement.
9. Adjust the occlusion with very fine diamonds or porcelain finishing burs.
10. Try to use a rubber dam for the entire seating process.

11. When doing multiple units you should try to seat all veneers at once. It's the best way to get them to fit together properly. Don't worry about getting cement stuck interproximally. It will break off within 7 days.

Veneers that require reduction can be temporized by using composite if your regular temporary material will not adhere. Follow these steps:

1. Do not etch your preparation, except for a small area in the center of the tooth!!! Simply place a little bonding agent in this small part of the facial of each tooth, then fill the tooth with composite.
2. <u>Dip your fore-ginger</u> in a little bonding agent and use it to flatten the composite on all of the teeth. The finger really works well for this. Shape the composite with your plastic filling instrument and cure it for 20 seconds a tooth. You can use matrix bands to separate the teeth if you desire, but this is not necessary as long as you do not let any composite get undercut into lingual embrasures and contacts. Instruct the patient to be careful chewing!!!

Your lab can also fabricate indirect temporaries, but they add too much to the cost.

Shade selection is critical. You must give your lab the shade of your preparations, as well as the final shade desired. I normally order A1 for all of my veneers. Your final shade, after luting, may be just slightly darker then you anticipated because the cements will darken a little after they set. Take this into consideration when matching single units.

YOU CAN NEVER BE LONELY AS LONG AS YOU HAVE IMAGINATION

Q & A

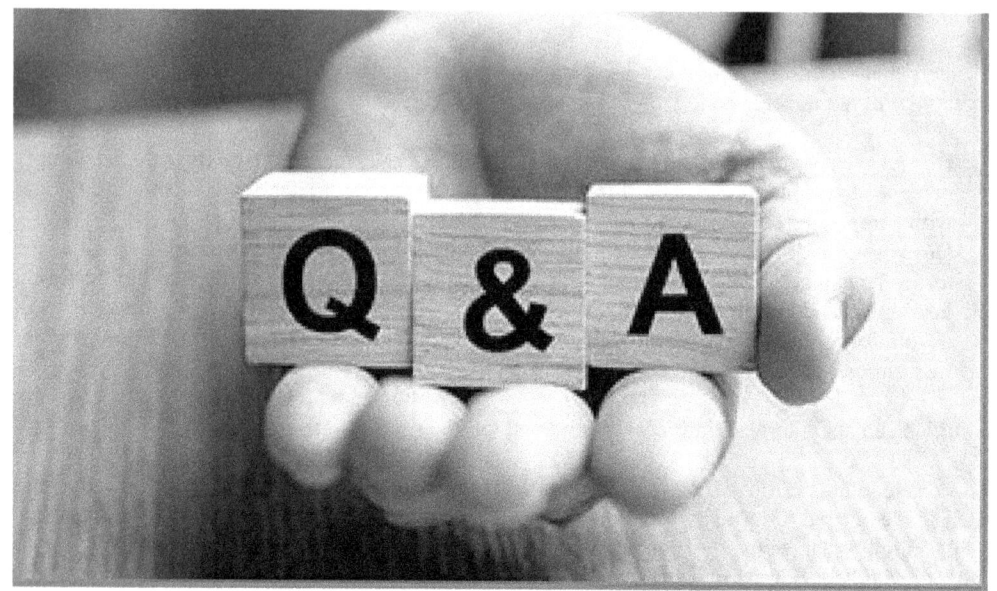

Q: You're recommending that we should accept managed care programs and capitation if we want to be busy, yet you also stress that we should maintain a low key, non-hurried schedule. How can we make any money seeing capitation patients and spending a lot of time with them?

A: First of all, you should never treat capitation and managed care patients if your chairs are full of fee-for-service patients. The reality of your situation, however, will quickly dictate your need to service segments of the population that established practitioners have no desire to treat. Take advantage of this by getting busy and practicing your clinical and communication skills. Sure you may have to work more than 40 hrs. per week to meet the demand, however the time that you will spend with each and every patient will pay off in the long term. You are not going to make a lot of money trying to provide quality care to capitation patients. However, the experience that you will gain through the ability to see more patients and perform lots of procedures will pay off in the long run. Don't cut short your approach just because you are seeing a lot of these patients. Develop your diagnostic abilities, practice your communication process, develop your case presentation approach, and improve your clinical speed and knowledge. Consider limiting your patient pool once your reputation speaks for itself and patients are willing to pay you for your expertise. The first five years of practice compromise a time in your career when you are not going to have a lot of choices about who you treat and what you treat. Use this to your advantage and stick to your guns.

Q: Should I try to improve my people skills or my clinical skills, during the first stage of my career?

A: That's like asking Henry Ford if he should have put the engine in the car before the tires. To be successful you must learn to balance all aspects of yourself. You won't get to do too much dentistry if you cannot educate and motivate your patients. Furthermore, if people don't like or trust you, you will be taking two steps forward and three back. If you are going to work in a high volume practice and your schedule will be dictated by people in three piece suits you may have a hard time practicing your case presentations and communication process. Again, stick to your Smith and Wesson. If you want to delegate some patient education to the assistants do so with your supervision and direction. I allow my assistants to perform a lot of patient education once I have had ample time to "bond" with that patient and develop rapport. But never shortcut your entire communication process. As far as clinical improvement goes, try to be the best you can be especially when it comes to being gentle and empathetic. Patients will refuse to see other dentists if you do not hurt them. They will follow you and be loyal. Also, the more procedures you perform the more you learn and the better you become at doing clinical dentistry. You will also decrease your re-makes and gain the knowledge that helps you to avoid unforeseen clinical circumstances and drawbacks. In other words, you will know which can has worms in it before you open it up. This will lead to better future diagnosis, faster procedural completions, and less complications.

Q: How can I spend so much time talking and educating my patients if I want to be profitable?

A: Again, at the sake of being redundant, you must develop rapport and gain patient trust. You cannot do so if you look in their mouths, study the x-rays, and make recommendations quickly. This is usually the standard of care in many high volume practices. If you want to build a quality, reputable practice, and career, you must get to know your patients by taking the time to listen to them and educating them. The actual basics of the clinical procedures and steps can be delegated to your assistants and to generic video-tapes. These professionally produced dental education tapes are also useful in motivating the patient and helping them comprehend dentistry through visualization. But the initial patient contact and relationship building must be done by you.

I am also a firm believer in not overdoing things and taking too much time with each patient. I like to stay busy and active during my daily schedule. Most patients do not require more than 15 minutes of your time during their initial visit. However, I will never compromise the need to build trust with new patients and get them to become a life-long friend, patient, and customer. Even if the patient does not need a lot of dental care I like to take the time to get to know them and welcome them into the practice. With comprehensive care patients I will normally take at least 30 minutes of my own time to explain their needs and the procedural requirements.

Therefore, new patients are scheduled for 45 minutes. They usually need either a simple cleaning, minor restorative and periodontal care, or more extensive treatment. I will not take more than five minutes to review their health history, x-rays, and perform a comprehensive exam. If the patient feels like talking, I listen. I will make mental notes of what they desire and center my findings around their perceived needs. My health history has a question that asks the patient what they feel is most important regarding their dental needs. This is the basis for my entire approach during the first visit.

If all they request is a simple cleaning then the hygienist or myself will quickly perform this, after the exam and x-rays. If the patient has unperceived needs then I will attempt to go into the education aspect. If they have periodontal problems there will obviously be no cleaning.

Most of the time, I will allow the assistant and hygienist to present brochures and play the appropriate educational videos that are specific for the patient's problems. I may go see another patient during this time, or I may decide to spend more of my time with the patient, if I feel that there is going to be extensive work and/or the patient is hesitant. If the patient needs a lot of work they normally get study models and another consultation appointment. If they have few needs, I try to get their cleaning finished and possibly even their minor restorative needs, before they leave. If the patient does not desire anything other than a cleaning I will make notes of their refusal for treatment and follow up in six months. If I have no time for minor restorative I will wait until their next recall and make a note in the computer to allow me a few extra minutes at that six month appointment.

Again, the key is to give yourself ample time to get to know your patients, while also being productive and efficient. That's why literature and videos are great for providing you with the flexibility to do other things, besides talk. Your actual patient contact time should not be longer than 15 minutes, except for your "large" cases. Allow your hygienist and assistants to help you build the patient trust. The hygienist is the pseudo-doctor and she is usually responsible for a lot of the rapport process in the office.

Q: You just spent a lot of time in this book on communication and patient education, yet you only spend a few minutes with each patient on this?

A: Yes, all of the material in this book does not need to be applied in an extensive manner. Sure it will be useful when doing large restorative cases and I do urge you to spend ample time with these patients. However, in a profitable practice economics do not allow for extensive bull-shitting sessions. Practice listening and addressing the patient's perceived needs, first and foremost. The remainder of your education will come easy once you have broken the ice and gained the patient's trust. During the early part of my career, I used to have a hard time presenting dentistry simply because I looked young and immature and patients did not have enough trust to spend a lot of their time and money in my care. I used to talk until I was blue in the face. I almost thought about getting a plumber's license at one point in time. As I build my reputation and skills I have reached the stage of my career where I no longer need to spend a lot of time tooting my horn and making recommendations. Patients know me, trust me, and respect me.

You will also find that many patients will not follow your recommendations during the early stage of your career. This is another reason that you need to see a larger number of patients than other established practitioners. I still treat patients for problems that I diagnosed five years ago. There is nothing more beneficial to your career than telling a patient what will happen with their teeth if they do not follow your advice. When that deep caries hits the nerve, and the patient wakes up at 2 a.m., guess who's advice they will remember?

The moral of the story is to not give up on educating your patients and diagnosing optimal dentistry. You will obviously have to spend a few more minutes with each patient than I do, because you simply have not encountered and treated tens of thousands of patients like I have. After five or seven years, you will find that your "shoot-the breeze" sessions will diminish in length and you will spend less time talking.

If you have an intraoral camera your patient education becomes very simple.

Q: I do everything possible to educate my patients and inform them of their needs, yet my case acceptance is poor and patients fail to show up for their appointments. What am I doing wrong?

A: Read this whole book again (ha, ha). Your patients are missing their appointments most likely because they cannot afford the care, or you have not met their emotional needs. Obviously, if you have not taken the time to explain to them how gentle your care will be than you can't expect them to overcome their hesitations. If you have not done a treatment plan than you can't expect them to know what to expect at each and every visit. If you have not received case acceptance than you have failed to gain the patient's trust, or you have missed one of the other points just discussed. You must get in the habit of achieving patient commitment before they schedule their next appointment. If the patient is not committed to treatment, and they do not appear excited about optimal care, than you will have a no-show. Never be afraid to ask the patient if they can afford the treatment presented. I routinely tell all of my new patients, *" I realize that this is a lot of money and I have discussed all of the consequences of not getting this work done with you. If you are determined to proceed with this work we can begin at your next visit and we can discuss how much each of your visits will cost. We will start with whatever you feel is most important. Is there any reason that may prevent you from getting this work done?"* You can offer alternative, low-cost treatment but be very careful when doing so. If you know that a tooth needs a root canal don't play David Blaine. You can use composite for many temporary restorative needs, but educate the patient in terms of drawbacks.

Remember, get patient commitment and meet their emotional needs!

Q: How much money should I be making during the first five years of my career?

A: According to the ADA, about as much as a plumber. That's the hard, cold truth. I think you should worry more about developing your personal and clinical skills during this stage. The money will come later. The world is thirsty for professionals who are experts at their trades, and are willing to provide quality above all else. Become a C.E. junky and practice, practice, practice. Start worrying about your financial indicators after five years. Learn to diagnose and treat the mouth as a whole, and not as single teeth. You will do more dentistry and you will do it better, faster, and more profitably.

Q: How should I get paid if I am an associate and I work at two different places?

A: Obviously, you need to hire yourself a good accountant. Ask your local society to refer some of these professionals that work with doctors and dentists. Incorporate if you feel that it is beneficial to your situation. Remember that you will be billing in your name for all of the patients that you see. It is helpful to use a Tax I.D. # for this process. Also, ask your accountant if it is necessary to write to the IRS each and every year if you are being paid a percentage of your collections and you still use your individual name to bill for the patient services. In other words, if you bill out $400,000 worth of services in your name and social security # and you get paid about $300,000 from the insurance companies than the IRS will think your income was $300,000. Your employer may only pay you $100,000 of this money collected (30% of $300,000). You may raise a red flag at the IRS because your individual income tax return will only show $100,000, yet all of the insurance carriers have reported $300,000 of income to the IRS on your behalf. Your accountant will need to address this issue. If you are in a group practice you may enjoy the ability of using the group practice tax I.D. # and name for all of your billing. You may also be hired as an employee and receive a paycheck with all taxes and deductions performed automatically for you. You still need to be careful when using your name for billing. My recommendation is that you set up your own Subchapter-S corporation. See your accountant!!!

Q: Should I learn about implants and orthodontics?

A: Yes, as a general overview. If you want to specialize and perform only implantology or orthodontics than think about graduate school. However, trying to be the jack of all trades will diminish from your ability to treat more patients with bread and butter dentistry. It will take away from your schedule. During the first five years I don't believe you should learn any specialty work. Implants are profitable if you plan on receiving referrals and limiting your practice to them. Otherwise, by the time you learn to place them, and restore them, you will have lost in other areas. Get your oral surgeon to do them. Make friends with your prosthodontist and have him/her restore them. But learn to offer them to your patients and make them a part of your treatment plans. Always offer implants before you offer fixed bridges! The same is true for orthodontics. I don't believe any general practitioner should be doing orthodontics, unless they decide to limit their practice to that. It takes a lot of continuing education to be able to perform orthodontics appropriately. Obviously you need to do a lot of it to be good at it. Get good at the bread and butter stuff, first.

Q: It seems as though esthetic dentistry is the future. How should I improve my skills in this area?

A: Hogwash! Bread and butter dentistry is still going to be the wave of the future. Ask yourself how many of your patients are willing to pay above $900 for a veneer? The answer is: not too many! Don't be brainwashed by all of the self-claimed experts who preach cosmetic care above all else. There are not too many practices in this country that can limit themselves to porcelain and composite. It's usually only the practices of these seminar speakers that can afford to limit their patient base to such work, and their income comes from the "speeches." Learn the basics and then worry about providing these services.

Q: Should I hire a financial adviser to handle my portfolio?

A: I am a strong believer in the do-it-yourself methods. With financial giants like Fidelity it is so easy to manage your own money. Financial advisers are usually just glorified representatives of their respective companies. Watching your own portfolio is the best way to go. Stick to mutual funds that invest in the basics of food, shelter, and entertainment. If you decide to use an investment firm you should realize that you will be limited to mostly the investments that the company makes extra commissions on. If you want to let a "pro" handle your money, I suggest that you hire a non-biased, non-partisan expert who has no interest in any investments. Remember: your practice and your profession is your #1 investment!

Q: What should I purchase first, an intraoral camera or laser?

A: Both

Q: How do I know what new products are good to use?

A: Remember that most dental products are the same basic chemicals packaged differently by the various manufacturers. Don't mix and match between manufacturer products because the formulations are slightly different. Don't ever rush to be the first to use a new product. Allow others to test the waters. Stick to traditional care whenever possible and allow time for inventions to prove themselves before you use them. Get your local supply salesman to provide you with literature on new products. Call the technical support lines of the manufacturers and quiz them about the chemical formulations.

Q: How do I build a quality practice and get more new patients that care about their teeth?

A: Let your fingers do the walking. Your reputation will spread like wild-fire once people get to know and trust you. If you are gentle, compassionate, skillful, knowledgeable, and pleasurable than people will seek your services. Don't hurt people, get them to trust and like you, and provide quality dental care. It's really not that complicated! If you are opening your own practice from scratch allow at least 3 years of development before you can see some returns. Learn about effective marketing and becoming your own consultant.

Q: It seems as though the practice that I work at has a high employee turn-over rate and astronomical payroll distributions. What could be the problem?

A: Lack of personnel management and inefficiency. Call our office or get outside help!

Q: How do I find qualified employees that don't cost an arm and a leg?

A: About the same way you can find a new Mercedes for $10,000. Steal it! I am a firm believer when it comes to not hiring employees with previous experience in the dental field. Most of my employees have worked either at a fast food restaurant or at a store in the mall. Seek employees that are working hard jobs for little wages. Visit your mall and fast food restaurants. Hire and train these employees. You'll be surprised how fast anyone can learn to do the tasks in your office. Obviously you need to develop your own customized training program. Our full dental office management program covers this topic at length.

Q: What seminars should I go to?

A: AGD, ADA, and state society meetings are the best bank for your buck. Take a weekend off and go absorb. There are few seminars that I attend any more, personally, because I can read most of this stuff for free in the monthly journals. Try to take hands-on participation courses whenever possible. Also, have a discriminating taste when you select your seminars. Many speakers are simply just full of hot air. My best mentors over the years have been local practitioners who are doing and not talking.

Q: What are your antibiotic choices?

A: Amoxicillin as my first choice. EES if allergic to penicillin. Augmentin for serious infections. Add 250 mg. of Flagyl if the infection has been stagnant for a few years, and/or there is cellulitis involved. Tetracycline or Doxy. for perio. ZPak for Amox allergy.

Q: How about pain medications?

A: Knock out the pain before it starts!!! T3 or Norco. For "trouble" patients: tell them you don't have a license to prescribe anything stronger than Norco. Four Advils also work great for most basic, non-invasive procedures.

Q: I get a lot of mail offering me quick ways to get rich and make money in my spare time. What's up with these?

A: Fly-by-nights. If anything is too good to be true than why would anyone tell you about it?

Q: Should I attempt to perform periodontal care and oral surgery?

A: Yes, yes, yes. But only after you have referred a few difficult cases to your local specialist and have had the opportunity to see the surgery first hand. Monkey see, monkey do. I did not do my first periodontal flap surgery until I watched ten quadrants performed by a local periodontist. It's not brain surgery! I would suggest that you do refer your full bony, and maybe even your partial bony impactions, especially if you have a larger than normal size patient.

Q: I spend a lot of time adjusting my crowns. What shall I do?

A: Spend more time on the temporary and the impression technique.

Q: I still get a lot of post-op sensitivity. What could I be doing wrong?

A: If you have taken care not to burn your tooth during preparation the only other major deal is to make sure that you have sealed the dentinal tubules. I seal all of my non-root canaled teeth. If your dentin is sealed you should have practically no post-op sensitivity. This comes in handy when doing crowns on vital teeth. Remember that a sealed tooth looks glossy after curing. If the tooth is not glossy add some more layers of primer and use a little moisture to 'drive' the primer into the dentinal tubules. Also remember that astringents can cause hyperemia in the pulp if you leave them on too long. Astringent should never stay in contact for more than 30 seconds with the tooth. It is as bad as leaving your etch on. They're both acids! Don't leave acids on the tooth!!! In conclusion, use lots of water irrigation during preparation, etch for no more than 20 seconds, and seal the dentinal tubules. Go back and read Chapters 26 and 27. Also don't forget to use 50:50 solution for disinfecting the tooth.

Q: Brochures can cost a lot of money. Which ones should I buy and from where?

A: Plenty of videos on Youtube. Desktop record them and play them on your computers in the clinic.

Q: I run into difficult situations when I treatment plan an amalgam/composite and the tooth ends up needing a root canal. Any suggestions?

A: With experience you will learn to diagnose the possible need for endo more often than not. Any large deep amalgam has the possibility to turn into a root canal. Any cavity that has penetrated the dentin has the same chance. Prepare for it. Make it a part of your consent and complication of treatment explanation. Treatment plan it as secondary treatment.

This question segways into another concept: that all patients should receive more care than expected. What I mean is the opposite of what you think. Prepare for the root canal, but do the restoration. Another great practice builder is as follows: if you quote a $2000 fee to a patient, finish the work for $1500 and donate the other $500 to a family member for their dental needs (or charity of their choice). Deliver more than you promise. Underpromise and overdeliver!!!

Prepare for the worst and give patients more than they thought they were going to get.

Q: Do you guarantee your work?

A: Always, and I tell my patient about the warranty. Composites for three years, crowns/bridges for fire years, partials/dentures for one year. The warranty is good only if their complete dental needs are finished as presented and they come back for their six month recalls. Alternative treatment is the patient's responsibility. Root canals will be re-treated if I missed something or filled improperly, within 3 years, and the final restoration has been completed. I have had only one re-treat in the last 10 years.

Get in the habit of letting your patients know about your guaranteed workmanship. If you know what you are doing you will never have to re-do your work. And I do mean, NEVER! Almost, never, that is! Patients won't believe that a dentist is guaranteeing their work. It's a great practice builder.

Q: Have you found anything useful to repair broken porcelain and metal facings?

A: If you want to TRY to repair these problems remember that you must etch the porcelain with HF acid, not phosphoric. The phosphoric is to be used only for etching enamel, removing the smear layer from the dentin, and to some degree etching metal. Let the HF acid sit on the porcelain for five minutes, not 20 seconds. Likewise, leave the phosphoric on the metal for at least five minutes. It is a good idea to use a Danville microetcher before etching. This helps to "clean" the surface. Follow the long etching with the Etch-Free from Parkell. After the Etch-Free use Parkell's Meta-Bond System, followed by your favorite bonding agent, curing, and then restoring with composite. Relieve the occlusion and you may have a chance of making the repair last at least a few weeks. Better yet, take out your guarantee and re-do the restoration. Ask yourself why the porcelain broke. Did you evaluate the occlusion closely???

Q: I have no luck getting paid for porcelain inlays. Have you heard of any way to get reimbursed for these?

A: Stick your head in a jar of pickles and blow hard. Most insurance programs will reimburse at the expense of an amalgam. Consider doing composites and charging your patients the difference!!! If you are determined to keep doing porcelain inlays for your MODs than you should get reimbursement from your patients. However, have you thought about the need to be "protecting" some broken cusps? You will find it easier to get payment if you document cuspal protection needs secondary to fracture. If a cusp is fractured the tooth needs some sort of full coverage. Dental insurance contracts are designed to reimburse crowns for fractured teeth. Don't document weak tooth anatomy or gross decay. <u>Document the broken cusps and the need for cuspal protection</u>. Ask for payment for the equivalent of a gold onlay. You will have a hard time proving to consultants that MOD restorations require more than an amalgam. The contracts are not written for this type of reimbursement. Don't fight it.

Q: Don't you think it's easier to do full flap surgery along with scaling instead of separating the procedures?

A: I guess if you had a headache you would want to try a few Tylenols before going to the brain surgeon. Just kiddin'! I like to be aggressive during my scaling and often I will do a lot of curretage and gingivectomy without flapping. Flaps should wait for primary healing. Flaps are a last resort. However, be aggressive during scaling and give the gums a chance to heal. You will be surprised that 99% of your periodontal cases will not need any further surgery. Don't forget subgingival irrigation and Doxy, Peridex! Laser is a must!

Q: How often do you work out and what kind of supplements do you take?

A: The key is not frequency but quality. I jog at least three times per week, followed by weightlifting and back strengthening. No more than 90 minutes. Two days per week I take karate lessons, including kick-boxing and stretching. I consume absolutely no soft drinks and I enjoy gulping at least a gallon of water per day. When I feel tired I drink water! I watch all fatty foods and try to avoid anything that is fried. If it looks saucy I stay away from it. I supplement my diet with medical grade herbs and vitamins because I offer holistic dentistry in my practice and I do BodyScan technology for health improvement. Most grocery foods have poor nutritional value. Seek a health food grocery store near your house. Read some books on this topic. It will change your life. And don't forget to get plenty of sleep and relaxation. Life is short.

Q: Why do so many dentists burn-out? Why do so many dentists struggle to make ends meet?

A: Lack of self motivation, I guess. While I look forward to dealing with problems and difficulties others avoid them and get withdrawn. They lose self-respect, motivation, and energy. Your mind can overcome everything. Better yourself with motivational books, tapes, and videos. Develop a positive frame of mind and learn to deal with negative things in your life. That which does not kill, teaches! Be decisive, blame yourself before others, be bold and courageous, take good care of the ones you love, be honest, be persistent, be forgiving, be decisive.

If you want to be successful develop a circle of friends that have the same views and goals in life. Visit dentists who are doing what you would like to do. Learn from them, emulate them, and become better than them. Stay away from losers and talkers. Stick around achievers and optimists.

Q: You make it sound so easy when it comes to writing down your goals and achieving them. I think it's getting harder and harder today to achieve what I want.

A: Only if you limit yourself. Remember the essence of time-frames and the concept of not trying to become an overnight success. Goals take time. But first, you must have them.

Q: How can I figure out my overhead when I am much slower clinically than more experienced dentists?

A: Do the following. If you are just out of school, consider yourself four times slower than senior dentists. After three years you will be about half as slow. After five or six years you will be about as fast as possible. This is one reason that I try to persuade recent graduates out of opening up their own practices. When you have more associates to share the same overhead you can compensate for the slow hands. Obviously you can also compensate through extended hours, but be careful about burning out. Worry about doing things right rather than doing them fast. The money will come!

Q: I have a hard time getting my assistant to get proper x-rays? What shall I do?

A: Take them yourself while she watches. Train your staff!!! Never perform a complete exam without proper x-rays. Check the distals of the cuspids! Evaluate the level of the crestal bone! Check out the adequacy of the root canals! Criticize the crown margins! GET PROPER X-RAYS. Without blueprints you will not have the chance to perform because you will not get the chance to diagnose. Don't shortcut yourself.

Q: How do I learn more about the kind of stuff in this book?

A: Look forward to one of our upcoming newletters. You will be informed!

FOR MORE INFORMATION ABOUT OUR COMPREHENSIVE DENTAL OFFICE MANAGEMENT PROGRAM PLEASE VISIT:

www.dentalofficemanagementprogram.com

DR JOHN'S TOP TEN LIST

Why Dentists Refuse To Be Succesful:

#10. Thinking that insurance will go away

#9. Referring too much out

#8. Not having patient friendly hours and policies

#7. Spending money on external advertising without looking in their backyard

#6. Allowing their high school graduate office workers too handle the money aspects of their business

#5. Thinking that marble floors and custom cabinets will sell expensive treatment plans

#4. Attempting to run a business without knowing all aspects of managing and coordinating that business

#3. Thinking like doctors and not businesspersons

#2. Believing that recalls and hygiene are more profitable than new patients and wet gloves

#1. Not realizing that new patients are the profit center of the practice

Need more info about our programs:

dentalofficemanagementprogram@gmail.com

www.ingramcontent.com/pod-product-compliance
Lightning Source LLC
Chambersburg PA
CBHW060827220526
45466CB00003B/1013